Better than Before Completely Healing and Enhancing My Brain

BETTER THAN BEFORE COMPLETELY HEALING AND ENHANCING MY BRAIN

an Autobiography

CATHY ANN GAFFNEY

Brain Phoenix TM

**DEDICATED TO
JANET (TEX)
LEAHY**

CONTENTS

DISCLAIMER

This book contains the experiences, views, and opinions of the author drawn from her recovery from traumatic brain injury and other events. It is intended to be inspirational, and while the book addresses the author's own recovery process from traumatic brain injury and other health threats and issues, the book is not engaged in rendering medical, mental health, or any kinds of professional services and advice. This book is not intended to substitute for the advice of competent professionals. The author disclaims any and all responsibility for any liabilities, loss or risk, personal or otherwise, which may be incurred, directly or indirectly, based on the use or application of any of the contents of this book. The reader should consult his or her medical, mental health, or other competent professional before attempting any exercise and recovery method including without limitation any specific forms or practices described in this book. The information contained in this book is offered without warranty or representation.

No portion or the entirety of this book may be reproduced, transmitted, or otherwise distributed in any media or by any means without the express written permission of the author.

ACKNOWLEDGEMENTS

Janet (Tex) Leahy, Robert N. Bowen, Richard Gaffney, Arlene Garvey, Rich Gaffney, Anne Baldwin, Susan E. Keenan, Chuck Lawhead, Paul C. Smith, Vicki Buck, Sonia Kirby, and Gus Spheeris.

Linda Browning, Brian Morris, Elizabeth Sinclair, Benjamin Brown, Francis Cottingham-Kelly, Karen Tracy, and Susan Bateman.

PART 1

1

FOREVER FALLING JANUARY 1989

I am two stories high, standing on scaffolding reaching onto the roof. The next moment I'm forever falling in a cool mist of huge, billowy soft clouds. The most perplexing sight is my boots overhead – they're a darker color. I wake up in an ambulance and scream in agony. Desperately, I try to get my bearings. I feel like a truck ran over me, backed up, and dumped the entire contents of the earth on top of me. I look down to see if all my body parts are connected. I appear to be in one piece, but am I paralyzed? I'm too scared to move. What happens if my legs don't work? I stare at my feet for what seems like a lifetime. Gathering my courage, I take a deep breath and close my eyes. With all the determination I can muster, I move my right toe and wiggle my feet. I'm beyond relieved, but it's short-lived.

In my brain, there's an electrical storm of faulty circuits exploding in every direction. Why can't I think right? How come my skull feels like it's going to split wide open, and my brain is going to burst through at any moment? I'm not paralyzed, but why am I still forever falling? What the heck is going on? I ask the paramedics what happened; my words come out scrambled. They look at each other with great concern. Now, I'm really scared. The paramedic's question stuns me. "Cathy, you don't remember?" I try to say no, but I sound like a little, little kid. They tell me the scaffolding collapsed, and I fell two stories.

The next moment the lights go out, and I continue plummeting in this forever fall. I wake up in the hospital with a whirl of doctors and nurses frantically working above me. They keep asking me over and over again, "Cathy, what happened? Do you remember what happened?" "Cathy, stay with us! Cathy, stay awake!"

All I want to do is sleep and easily drift off. In a drowsy state, I feel myself being gently placed into a warm, relaxing ocean current. I know I'm alive, but I don't understand what's happening. Time passes, and I sense I need to wake up. I see an obscure figure waving me over to an exquisite sandy beach. This place feels like home, but it's not like anything I've experienced. Inside my gut I understand these words, yet no words are spoken; Have a seat Cathy; relax in the warmth of the sun and enjoy the *beautiful* ocean. As the word *beautiful* is communicated, it's like these arms open up and lovingly welcome me home.

I look all around. I seem to be alone, yet I still sense an extraordinary loving presence. I don't understand what's happening. My thinking is crystal clear, I am completely free of pain, and I have a sense of calmness within and around me. I can only describe this as Love with a capital "L." However, the word Love does not even come close to expressing this profound, pure sense of Unconditional Love. Some might call it God, Buddha, Allah, or a Higher Being etc., though in this place, words are insignificant.

I stretch my legs and sink my cold toes into the silky warm sand which warms me from the inside out. Without any words, I experience the profound simplicities of Love, life, and the connections between us all. Love is the only thing that matters. Either I am choosing to move forward, in and towards Love by growing, changing, and fully living life. Or, I am choosing to travel backwards, barely existing, and withering in fear. Each moment, I make a decision and take actions about how I live my life and the direction I am traveling in and towards. I have this sense in my gut that I need to make a decision.

I take in a deep breath and decide to continue being a positive person and to become my true authentic self. At once, this expansive Love fills me. I relax and soak in what I can only describe as *paradise*. My entire being, from the inside out, is connecting with this Love which is in everyone and everything. For the first time in my life, I am my true essence; I am bliss.

Surveying the emerging panorama, the vibrancy and light is almost too much to experience; it is perfection. I have been searching outside myself for this feeling, this pure Love and connection. The last place I thought to look was *inside*. I want to stay here forever; then, I hear distant voices as I move between two worlds. "Cathy, stay with us!" "Cathy, you're going to be okay." I am on a threshold.

The next moment, I'm back in the ER with all the medical people above me. A nurse leans towards my face and says. "You're going to be okay; we need you to stay awake." On the inside I'm smiling, yet I'm in massive pain. I try to say that I want to go home and I want to go to sleep. Again, I'm shocked to hear this little, little kid's voice coming from me.

I notice something strange as I observe the people above me. Inside my body, I'm aware of all this ramped-up energy flying all over the place; it's exuding from the people working on me. Most of the doctors and nurses are calm, focused, and have my best interest at heart. Although they keep telling me that I'm going to be okay – their words don't match their energy. People's truths are revealed through this energy that's exuding from inside and around them, not their words. A few of the professionals are afraid and doubt their medical abilities. They're desperately trying to hide their fears and want to treat me as quickly as possible to avoid being exposed. One person seems totally disinterested. It's like I've interrupted his break, or maybe he just wants to move on to the next crisis. I don't understand what's happening. My brain isn't working right, my body is broken, yet I'm having these lucid insights from *deep inside my body*. Why don't people's energies match their words? How come they don't they say what they really mean, and what the heck is this energy and *inner awareness*?

The next moment, I am given a choice between two worlds. Either, I exist in this excruciating pain with a muddled brain and busted body. Or, I live in the paradise of Love – Real Love. Before I can answer, I am filled with Love, gazing at and I am one with this magnificent ocean. Slowly, I take a deep breath and gently exhale. I am free, and everything is right in the world and within me. My head is lucid, my vision is clear, and there is no pain. I savor each moment. *I am home*! There's a feeling, an emerging light. Love and peace draw me; then, I am being pulled back.

Someone speaks, "Cathy, stay with us!" Oh God, I'm in so much pain and utterly confused. My head is so full; it feels like my brain is going to explode out my skull. I ask to go home, but I sound dimwitted. The doctors look at each other in disbelief. I must be in really rough shape.

People think broken bones are the worst of my problems, time will heal them. No one has any idea of the severity of my injuries. I'm more like Humpty Dumpty who has fallen from the wall and landed with a broken body and a scrambled brain. Even though I know I physically hit the ground, busting my body and brain, I don't understand why I continue forever falling in this cool mist with my boots overhead?

THE THICK, BLURRY GLASS PRISON IN MY BRAIN

I despise hospitals and don't understand why I have to stay here. My friends explain that I have a lot of broken bones on the right side: clavicle, wrist, a lot of ribs in my back, and my head hit the pavement big time. There's also major bruising everywhere. I move ever so slightly and pain shoots through me. My body feels like it's crunching inside. Although I'm frustrated, the hospital stay is a little easier with all my visitors. People swap stories about how much fun we had at the beach on weekends, hanging out eating ice cream, and watching the parade of people walk by on summer nights. I don't remember, and I'm not able to follow their vibrant conversations. Some people I know, while others I don't recognize; they're friendly, but unfamiliar. A cold shiver runs through me as I try to remember – my mind is blank. Is this a nightmare? If it is I want to wake up. I want my life back.

People begin to notice problems with my memory, speech, and overall brain function. As another group of visitors leaves, a man walks in and they exchange hugs. The man stands in front of the bed and talks with me as a friend. Inside, I sense he cares deeply about me, but I don't know him. A few minutes later his energy changes; then, a look comes over his face as he asks if I know who he is. With every ounce of willpower I can muster, I try to wade through the dense sludge in my brain. Obviously, he knows and loves me, but he is a stranger. Dejectedly, I hang my head. He quickly leaves, and my body begins to tremble.

I'm imprisoned inside my brain by a thick, blurry glass wall. I turn to my left and touch the prison wall with both hands. Why is there a wall in my brain, and how come I'm able to touch it? I push; then, with all my might I pound on the prison wall with both fists. No matter how much I try, I'm not able to break through or even dent this seemingly impenetrable fortress. Why can I see and touch this wall in my brain, and why is it imprisoning me? Fear grips me. I'm locked in my own mind – completely disconnected from everything outside this prison, including my body. I can see my feet, but my brain doesn't know where my feet are.

The world I lived in my entire life is now a foreign outside world, and I no longer know how it works. From inside the thick, blurry glass prison in my brain, I'm looking out and alone as any human can be. The depth of loneliness and agony is unfathomable, yet there's also a little bit of peace. Though, the peace is paltry compared to the loneliness. At least in the solitary confinement of jail, people have a little interaction with the guards, but not inside my prison.

I have so many questions inside the prison in my brain, but I don't have the ability to speak them. I don't understand why the doctors and my loved ones aren't able to see me and help me escape this prison in my brain? How come I can't think right and remember? Why is it so difficult to get information into and out of this prison? I want to break through and connect with people and with my body, but I don't know how. Why doesn't anyone help me?

My brain has been stupefied, and I've become an inert observer of life. I struggle through this dense, murky inner world, constantly playing catch up as I watch life pass by. I feel like I'm watching a badly-dubbed movie with a distorted picture that keeps skipping and the sound turned up to an ear-splitting level. I look down at the cup of lime green stuff jiggling on my food tray and wonder. Is this what my brain is like now? No, this lime green stuff is too firm.

At any moment, it feels like my skull is going to burst open and what used to be my brain will explode and disintegrate into nothingness before it hits the wall. I grab my head to keep my skull intact, surprisingly there's a bit of relief. I let go and the pain roars back. There also feels like a ten-inch icicle is constantly being shoved into the inside corner of my left eye socket and deep into my brain. Slowly, I try to grab the icicle with my left hand, nothing is there. I press the tip of my left thumb directly into the inside eye socket; the pain slightly eases. I let go and grimace. Although my entire body is in pain, the constant, excruciating pain in my brain is unbearable.

Time passes, but I don't have a clue as to what day it is; I've lost the ability to tell time. I know its winter because people are wearing big coats, and there's a chill coming from the window to my right. Its okay that time no longer has meaning. In fact, I don't know why I ever let time have control over me.

The orthopedic doctor, a no-nonsense doc, walks in. He stands by my bed looking at the papers in his hand. In my broken speech I try to explain how I'm hovering above my body and won't come back into my body until the pain disappears. I realize what I'm trying to say is nuts, but the doctor's answer surprises and comforts me. He tells me that when people fall, they leave their body just before they hit the ground. He reassures me that I'm not crazy.

After ten confounding and pain-filled days, so people tell me, I leave the hospital to heal the traumas to my body. Physically, I'm incapable of taking care of myself, and move in with my partner. Over the next few weeks, she notices huge memory, speech, and fatigue problems. I've forgotten how to read, add simple numbers, cross a street, use the phone, and have lost most words, even simple ones. When I want something, I slowly point to it. Somewhere inside my brain I know I'm articulate, intelligent, vibrant, strong, athletic, and independent, yet I'm not able to make connections in my brain. Arrgh, this is beyond frustrating! How do I break through this thick, blurry glass prison in my brain?

More time passes. The weather is just beginning to change although it's still cold outside. My partner and I are invited to an afternoon potluck. We arrive, and she is excited to see our friends. All I want to do is sleep. I sleep eighteen hours plus a day, and I'm still plagued by crushing exhaustion.

I sit and watch the lively conversation and banter among our friends. I hunger to speak, yet I've got to travel through this thick pea soup to do it. My mouth opens and what little that comes out is jumbled. The conversation stops as everyone turns to look at me. There's an uncomfortable silence as I desperately search for words. I'm startled by the explosion of a fork as it drops and rattles on a plate. Utterly disoriented, I glance up and catch sight of the "look." The expression on my friend's faces is the same as the paramedics in the ambulance. There's also something new – a scent in the air which smells like fear. Does fear have a smell? Exuding from inside their bodies, and onto and into my chest is people's negative energy gunk; they're afraid. But, it's *my inner body that's aware and experiencing this, not my busted brain.* Are they scared of me, and what I've become? Or, are they afraid because they have to deal with me, and they don't know how? Someone breaks the tension and says, "You're okay Cathy; it's all in your head." Everyone laughs uncomfortably, including my partner.

The conversation continues without me; though, now there's a polite tension. Exuding from most people is fearful energy. Their smiles are strained, yet they're trying to talk upbeat. Why doesn't their energy match their words and outer selves? How come they're not taking responsibility for their energy and speaking their truth? Why are some people hiding behind walls? They have the ability to tear down their walls and be free; instead, they keep fortifying their walls. Yet, I don't have the ability to break through the prison in my brain?

Inside the thick, blurry glass prison, I have a new perspective. My busted brain is absolutely useless, yet *being aware of my inner body* continues to be enormously helpful in deciphering the foreign outside world. What is this *inner awareness?* Did I always have it and just didn't pay attention? I don't know, but this is my second big *inner awareness experience.* Are these inner awareness experiences a coincidence, or are they a clue to help me discover a way out of this prison in my brain? Again, I don't know.

On the way home, I fall asleep and drool from the relentless exhaustion. I climb into bed, but I'm not able to lift my legs. My partner takes off my shoes, and tucks me in. I am completely humiliated and too tired to care. Humiliation has become my normal existence.

A FAN IN THE FOREIGN OUTSIDE WORLD

My partner brings me to the bank to cash a check. While she runs a quick errand, I try to figure out what to do with the piece of paper she gave me. I look around and watch people walk over to a high desk in the middle of the room. Then, they go to the glass-walled area with smiling people on the other side. At the high desk, people have very serious faces. They're intently focusing on their papers while silently moving their lips. I try to mimic what they're doing with the papers, but they're way too fast. When they look up, their bodies are tight, and they seem anxious. Is it because I'm watching them? No, they don't see me; their fixated on their papers and the glass-walled area.

I watch them walk to the glass wall and follow what they do. When I push the paper through the opening, there's a rush of air that surprises me. The woman turns the paper over and brusquely states, "You didn't sign it." Her eyes squint, and her head turns slightly to the side. I look around to figure out what I'm supposed to do. I'm starting to sweat, and my heart is beating faster. I see the person next to me write on the tall end of the paper. I take a deep breath, my shoulders relax, and I scribble on the paper. She stamps the paper, and I sense a new energy, she seems annoyed. Then, I see a new expression, her body and face takes on a sort of I don't care kind of slump. She counts out the paper, spreading it into a fan shape.

I walk out the door with my new paper fan. My partner rushes towards me. She scolds me and tells me to put the money away. She looks around to see if anyone has noticed. When she calms down, she asks if I understood what happened. In my broken speech, I tell her that I didn't know what to do with the paper she gave me. Her energy changes to compassion; her body opens and her shoulders drop. How is it that my inner body is aware and knows what's going on, yet my brain is absolutely worthless? Although I still don't understand all of this, I need to keep focusing and developing the only thing that's working – *inner awareness*. My partner now understands the problem in my brain is more extensive than she thought. In a few months, she will end the relationship.

Before the accident, I could balance three bank accounts in my head. I figured complex carpentry math problems with ease, and I was an eloquent public speaker. Now, I sense I've fallen backwards into the world of a two-year old. I talk and look like a simpleton, and I've lost the ability to read, write, and add basic numbers. Trying to speak a simple two or three word sentence is beyond challenging, and the exhaustion is crippling. Every waking moment, I feel as if I've worked for seventy-two hours straight at extraordinarily hard manual labor, with only a five-minute break every eight hours. Life, as I knew it, has completely vanished. This is my new inner home – no *home* isn't the right word; I'm not supposed to be here. My home is out there – in the foreign outside world.

Rising, from somewhere deep inside, is a tremendous drive to be free, to be reconnected, and to get my life back. How do I break through this thick, blurry glass prison in my brain?

FROM A PERSON TO A PIECE OF PAPER

I'm staring out the passenger window looking down at Cape Cod Canal. It's another gloomy, cold day; though, the water and area far below are very beautiful. I'm looking forward to my appointment with one of the top neurologists at Beth Israel Hospital in Boston, a teaching hospital for Harvard Medical School. Hopefully, this doc will see me inside the prison in my brain and know how to break me out.

During the appointment, the doctor keeps asking really simple questions. The vast majority of the time I'm not able to answer even though I know some of the answers. I muster up every ounce of energy and speak a few more words than usually, but I'm not able to express what I really want to say. Again, the thick, blurry glass wall is preventing me from getting information in and out of my brain like I want to. There are all these disconnections in my brain, like something is blocking me. Inside, my brain, I am smarter than what comes out in their foreign outside world.

After a thorough examination, the doctor gives his diagnosis: maybe a brain injury (Traumatic Brain Injury; TBI), epilepsy, or merely a concussion. He prescribes an anti-seizure medication and sends me home. His parting words are, "Time will tell." I leave the doctor's appointment absolutely exhausted.

Shortly thereafter, I have a severe reaction to the medication and return to the hospital as an inpatient on the brain unit. In my scrambled brain, this is hilarious. I'm in the brain unit; they must think I'm smart!

Numerous times, I'm startled awake by ten or more doctors surrounding my bed. Inside, I'm very aware that while they want to help, it's more important to impress the head doctors and to outperform their fellow doctors. Their competition results in a polite elbowing match, without any body blows. Although Beth Israel Hospital is a wonderful facility, it will be my most impersonal medical experience. I am not a person; they treat me as just another piece of paper. Before the TBI, I was a highly functioning adult; people spoke *with* me. Now, most people speak *about* me. I feel like a chair – an inanimate object. Yet, I'm consumed with the memory of my former articulate, intelligent, vibrant, strong, athletic, and independent self.

During my hospital stay, I undergo many tests and examinations, including a Neuropsychological test (Neuro Psych test) to determine the extent of brain damage. After all the testing is complete, one of the doctors explains the results in her office. The doctor keeps talking and talking in this medical jargon that I don't understand, while I cringe in pain from the bright light from the huge window and florescent light overhead. I grab my skull to lessen the pain, the relief is miniscule. All I want to do is crawl out of her office and sleep.

The doctor keeps going on and on about these numbers, especially 68. What the heck is she talking about? Below 70 is what they label people as mentally retarded, and in my broken speech, I ask if this is what she means. Her answer shocks me. "Yes."

Time stops! I am completely stunned! There's a deafening silence in the room. I don't understand. How could my IQ drop? Inside, I'm aware the doctor is extremely distressed; her heart aches that she had to tell me this news, and compassionate energy is exuding from her. I look up – her energy matches her face and whole being. Her eyes are very sad as she leans forward. She hesitates to speak. How could it get any worse? I take a breath, and steady myself in the chair. I'm ready for anything she says. "There is no hope of recovery, ever."

The chair seems to give way, and plunges me even deeper into the cool mist of huge billowy clouds with my boots overhead. Her words reverberate off the walls and slap me in the face. *My IQ has dropped below the level of mental retardation and there's no hope of recovery, ever. Ever!*

I am in the depths of despair – imprisoned in my brain – lost and completely, utterly alone. I drag myself back to my room and sleep. Sometime later I wake up; as usual, the pillow is wet from my drool. Am I like those people with brain problems I've seen my entire life? Why are they still using such an archaic, degrading term to describe people with low IQ's in this day and age (1989)? I don't want to have this label or any label on me, nobody would. Why don't they come up with a better term? Rather than focusing on all the negatives of my test results, what the doctor said, and the way they label people, I decide to keep moving forward. I do not and will not accept their diagnosis and labels, or anyone's labels. Maybe the professionals at the rehabilitation hospital can put my scrambled brain back together again. While waiting to get into rehabilitation hospital, I return home, and I'm launched on a most interesting journey.

2

AN UNEXPECTED
BLESSING
IN AN UNOPENED
GIFT

From the bedroom window, I see people have shed their big, warm winter coats for lighter ones. The trees have tiny, bright leaves, and the grass is greening up. Inside my thick, blurry glass world, I tell time by the seasons, by what people wear, and by the weather. I rather like my new way of understanding time; it's natural and makes more sense. In the distance, I hear different construction projects; people are getting ready for the tourist season. Life is blooming in the foreign outside world while I remain shackled inside my brain. I miss working with wood and life as I knew it.

To keep my spirits up while waiting to get into the rehabilitation hospital, my friends take me out for different activities. Today we're at the beach. It's too cold to go into the water, though I'm enjoying sitting on the sea wall watching the ocean. I'm distracted by a young man walking towards me. He's looking directly at me, not at my friends. Who is he? I search and search my brain, but I don't know him. He gets closer, and *I have an inner awareness inside my body – a beautiful sensation of warmth and goodness which begins inside my chest and is moving into my abdomen. My entire inner torso is open, warm, and relaxed. This inner sensation brilliantly communicates the man's profound loving kindness and compassion for me, and how helpful he's been, especially recently. There are no words; it's an inner awareness – a knowing, and maybe that's why I missed it before.* Why is *my inner body aware* that he's been very kind, and has helped me greatly? Yet my brain is utterly void of any memories of who he is and what he's done?

He cheerfully says, "Hi Cathy!" Who is this man? He obviously knows me. I try to say what I'm experiencing inside my body but the words don't come out right. It takes me forever to sort of say in this little, little kid's voice "nice"; then, I point at him. His smile widens. Why can't I say a simple three word sentence, "You nice me" – which isn't even a sentence? I'm getting worse. Where are my words? I've lost my words. I try to say that I don't know how he's helped me. Again, the words come out jumbled. Inside, I'm grateful for the few people who sort of understand my broken speech and gestures. My friends and this man look at one another; then, back at me. Exuding from them is tender, loving kindness. I want to tug at one of my friend's shirt to ask who is this man, and what has he done, but my busted body hurts too much to move.

Finally, one of my friends shines some light on this very confusing situation. He explains that the man has given me rides to a physical therapy office which is about 45 minutes one way. He's also brought me food and has been an all around awesome human being. I breathe a sigh of relief as I hear the verbal confirmation of what my inner awareness has already revealed. How come my inner body absolutely knows this, yet my brain doesn't have a clue?

I struggle to thank the man for his kindness. Once again,

everyone looks at one another then back at me. Exuding from them and entering my inner body is pure love. Their bodies are open, and there's a warm energy exuding from them, as all of these wonderful loving words are being exchanged, yet no one is speaking. After a bit, people begin to talk. Although I'm not able to follow their energetic conversations, I'm grateful for the inner awareness experience of loving kindness being expressed, without words from one human being to another, and towards me.

I continue having inner awareness experiences with different people and situations. With most people my inner body is open, warm, and relaxed. However, when people don't have my best interest at heart, my inner body closes and becomes cold and tight. Just like a little kid, I try to hide behind one of my friends. Although I don't like the negative experiences, they too are developing my inner awareness which is guiding me, step by step, to understand who will help me and who will take advantage etc. out there in the foreign outside world. Though, I do have a blind spot when it comes to the people in my family, but that's a story for another day.

What I find fascinating about this whole *inner awareness* experience is I've been with my body 24/7 from the moment I was born. Yet, I didn't know my inner body responded to people and situations. It's like I've gone back to the bare basics of communication. Maybe what's happening to me is similar to someone who has lost their sight and their other senses compensate. Have I opened to this inner awareness of my inner body because my brain isn't working right, and my inner awareness has to take over? Maybe my inner body has always responded to people and situations, but I relied too heavily on my brain and didn't pay attention to my inner body. In some ways, learning this inner awareness skill is similar to being thrust into a foreign country without a language interpreter. However, inner awareness is more than learning a new language. To understand how the foreign outside world works; I need to become aware of how my inner body is responding, and the more I practice, the more my inner awareness improves.

A memory of an event trickles through the sieve in my brain and very, very slowly a connection is made. Remembering this is major because I've lost months of memory before the accident. Three weeks before the accident, I was abruptly awakened in the middle of the night. I sat up and looked around, everything was peaceful. Deep within, I experienced a gut sense or inner knowing, like a quiet whisper without words. This gut sense was warning me that it was dangerous to work on the roof at work, a project that would begin in three weeks. I had never experienced a gut sense, inner knowing, or still small voice, and had never really paid attention to my inner body. I certainly wasn't a touchy feely, new age type of person. I liked things to be tangible. Instead of paying attention to this very unusual experience, I went back to sleep.

In the morning, I woke up and thought I had had a bad dream and told myself to forget about it. At work, I kept telling myself that I was living my dream and being paid to do what I love; carpentry. But I couldn't shake the sense of impending danger. Every night the same warning woke me, except on Friday and Saturday nights. In hindsight, I believe I slept well on those nights because I wasn't going to work the next morning. At the end of each work day, as I was putting my tools in my truck, I gave myself a hard time for blowing things way out of proportion.

The next Sunday night, I was awakened again. This time my heart felt like it was going to explode out my chest. In my gut, there was an enormous sense of danger of working on the roof. The next morning, I got up the courage and asked the foreman if I could do another job rather than work on the roof. While I was speaking, four other employees gathered in back of me. When I finished, they told the foreman they too didn't want to work on the roof. Although it felt good not to be alone, I wish they had waited to say something after I got the okay to do another job. In no uncertain terms, the foreman told us that if we didn't work on the roof, we could find another job. It was January and for a carpenter to have steady work at that time of year was a blessing. In that moment, I made a decision which changed my life. Rather than have faith in myself that I would find another job. I chose to believe the lie that I could not find work because it was winter. In time, I will learn, when I believe a lie, I will always run smack into the truth.

The night before the accident I woke up in a complete state of panic. I couldn't breath and was drenched in sweat. My inner body was screaming at me not to go to that job site – again, without words. I didn't pay attention and my life was forever changed.

I sense there's a great significance with this memory and the inner awareness experiences: in the E.R., the potluck, the unknown caring, helpful man, and other experiences. Although I'm not sure what's happening, I do not want to repeat the same mistake as I did before the accident – it is vital to pay attention to my gut sense and develop my inner awareness. Maybe being aware of my inner awareness will help me break through the thick, blurry glass wall in my brain. But, how do I develop this inner awareness? I'm sleeping 18 hours a day, yet I'm still exhausted. This leaves little time or energy to work on developing my new inner awareness skill. Consciously, I make a decision – from this moment forward, I will trust what my gut is guiding me to do, because it would be nuts not to. Next, I get a strong gut sense to keep developing my inner awareness – I believe being aware of how my inner body responds will help me understand people and situations in the foreign outside world, and maybe more.

I laugh out loud. There's a lot more happening inside my brain than all their test results. Inside, I'm able to make decisions, create questions, reason, and make a plan. But, I'm not able to get much in and out of the thick, blurry glass prison. On the outside, I'm as dumb as a post and as slow as a snail. People think my light bulb has gone dim, but they don't know what's happening inside. Don't get me wrong, I know I've got major brain damage. Inside the thick, blurry glass wall, I know I'm not the sharp, intelligent, athletic person I used to be. But, inside I am smarter and sharper than their test results. Maybe someday people will develop tests that can penetrate the thick, blurry glass wall. Then, their test results will paint a more accurate picture of what's happening inside the brain. Unfortunately, future tests will not help me now.

I decide to change my perspective; *out of every negative situation have come many positive, healthy experiences and transformations because I've learned to be open, to look for, and to purposefully work for them.* Inside, I consciously set my focus; I will keep exploring and delving deeper into my inner awareness training. My hope is this inner awareness thing will help me discover a way to liberate myself from this prison in my brain and be reconnected.

****

[Heads Up Reader! This is very important, and it will be the only heads up in the book. My precise method Brain Phoenix ™, especially my inner awareness training was the key that unlocked the prison in my brain, completely healed and enhanced my brain, and fully reconnected me. All of my improvements occurred from the – inside out. First, as I step by step delved deeper into my inner awareness training, my abilities improved, bit by bit: mentally, physically, verbally, memory, energy, balance, etc.

In my brain healing journey it became crystal clear that trying to push intellectual knowledge and outside techniques through the thick, blurry glass wall did not work and was not the solution to completely heal and enhance my brain. Information is not transformation. This analogy helped me to put this into perspective. If an engine is clogged or running rough, or a computer is slow; I wouldn't add more fuel into the engine, or download more information or videos into a computer and expect the problem to be fixed. It's the same with the brain. Inputting more outside, intellectual information and techniques into a busted brain and expecting it to break through the thick, blurry glass prison did not work. What's interesting is when I focused on outside techniques and outside success I always floundered and got off course.

As you continue reading my brain healing journey, please keep in mind that there wasn't a guide or map...not even a pamphlet to show me how to free myself from the prison in my brain. I was on my own. While I was developing my method I experienced great success and a few missteps, and I learned from both. A journey doesn't always mean traveling in a straight line. I also faced obstacles, and as with every human being the biggest ones are inside. I found ways to persevere even when I didn't want to or thought I could. Humor and a positive mind-set were two of the tools that helped me to enjoy my journey and created momentum. My most vital technique – my inner awareness training and my precise method Brain Phoenix ™ guided me, step by step, in my brain healing journey. The reason for this Heads Up is in the past, and even as I publish this book, there is the mind-set that it is impossible to heal the brain. My hope is you will have an open mind. I believe the only place impossible resides is in the mind, but not in mine, and hopefully not in yours. My journey continues.]

THE
REHABILITATION
HOSPITAL
JULY 1989

My favorite time of year is summer; I absolutely love warm weather. I've just celebrated my birthday, and I am really grateful to be going into New England Rehabilitation Hospital (N.E.R.H.). Hopefully, they can wake me from this nightmare.

At rehab, I have an exceptional team of doctors, nurses, neuropsychologists, speech, physical, occupational, and more therapists than I can remember. For the first time since the TBI, I'm surrounded by people who understand me and my broken speech. They look me *in* the eye, and talk *with* me as a person, not as a piece of paper. I sense this is more than a profession for them; they want the very best for their patients. When I'm around most of them, my inner body is open and warm. Step by step, it's getting a little easier to delve deeper into my inner awareness training – how my inner being responds to people and situations, which is helping me to better understand how the foreign outside world works.

The head of my team is Dr. Peterson. She's the first doctor, since the TBI, who treats me as a fellow human being. She looks directly at me, talks with me, and listens intently. She seems to spend extra time with me; even though, it's the same amount of time as other doctors' appointments. Maybe it's because she's present. Inside, I sense a great strength, calmness, and compassion exuding from Dr. Peterson.

Extensive therapies and tests are ordered, including another neuro-psych test, which takes eight hours to complete. To compensate for my extreme fatigue, the test is broken down into smaller sections. In between all the testing, I have numerous therapy sessions. I really appreciate that patients at rehab are treated with respect, kindness, and understanding. However, even in this wonderful facility, there are a few people who treat the paper, not the person.

One day, I'm between therapy appointments, resting in my room. A young doctor, whom I've never seen before, walks in and stands above me. He's intently reading and flipping the pages on my chart. While reading he's speaking in this medical jargon that I don't understand.

Inside I'm aware that he's all closed up, but he doesn't have bad energy. I figure he's either trying to be an ultra-distant professional or he's aloof. I also sense that he doesn't know how to handle me and this situation. I realize he hasn't made eye contact. Is he trying to protect himself? I decide to verbally engage him to the best of my ability. He persists in his total focus on everything else, except me. Once again, I've become invisible. His disrespect is absolutely frustrating. Why doesn't he look at me? I gather all my strength, sit up, and put my face right next to the chart. Now, he has to see me. He glances my way, but looks right through me; then, he quickly looks away. I sigh. Another medical professional who treats the paper, not the person. Will I ever be seen again?

A few days later, Dr. Peterson walks into my room; her energy is completely different, anger is exuding from her. Something must be very wrong because she's usually calm, cool, and collected. Is she mad at me? A few seconds later, the young doctor trails her; this time his head is hung low. Dr. Peterson greets me; then, she stands beside the head of my bed, facing the young doc and myself. The young doc sits in the chair beside my bed, faces me and once again speaks his medical jargon. Even if I had an intact brain, I don't think I could understand him. I look at Dr. Peterson; she's staring intently at the young doc and inwardly fuming. This very intelligent man doesn't understand the simplicities of human interaction. His attempt at an apology for how poorly he treated me is sorely missing the mark.

When he finishes speaking, Dr. Peterson asks me questions, about how the young doctor dealt with me. I try to answer, but I don't have my words. I try to remember a word the nice rehab professionals use to describe people's poor behavior. I know the word begins with a "P," but I don't remember the word. Finally, sounding like a little, little kid, I say "P" and sort of get out "word." Dr. Peterson with a really quizzical look on her face asks, "Patronized?" I point to her, and nod my head up and down while trying to express that he didn't look at me. Dr. Peterson continues prompting me with questions, but again I don't have my words. Where are my words?

The conversation ends as quickly as it began. Dr. Peterson who's still totally peeved, walks out the door; her energy and the look on her face is – no one on my watch disrespects my patients! The young doctor follows her, with his head hung low, shoulders slouched, and eyes glued to the floor. This experience reminds me of a principal who's just schooled an unruly student.

I lie back in bed, and try to make sense out of what just happened. How did Dr. Peterson hear about the situation with the young doc? I don't know. I've also never seen a doctor get in trouble over the treatment of a patient; this is an extraordinary event. For the first time since the accident I rest easy; a medical professional is in my corner. Dr. Peterson has my back.

I'm told that weeks have passed, and the testing process at rehab is complete, for now. A family meeting is scheduled where my entire team will present their findings. The meeting takes place in a tiny, dimly-lit office. I'm elbow to elbow with all the therapists, specialists, and doctors who've been so very kind to me. One by one, each professional speaks candidly about my extensive brain problems, treatment plan, and expectations. What little I can follow is devastating to hear.

My short-term memory is decimated. My math, reading, and verbal skills are practically non-existent. I've forgotten how to use everyday items: a phone, a watch, a hand screwdriver, a stove and oven to name just a few. I don't understand. I'm a carpenter; why don't I know the name for pencil, or how to use a hand screwdriver? This is beyond frustrating. *Do I have to learn everything all over again?* In time, I'll learn that my left temporal lobe, the verbal center, is decimated, and I believe they say there is also some damage in my frontal lobe and brain stem. After three therapists have given their report, I stop listening – the truth is too hard to bear. I stare at the floor as people speak about me and my condition.

Inside the prison in my brain, I decide to take stock of other things. Distraction and fatigue are huge problems. A gnat has better focus than I. At the slightest noise, I completely lose focus. I'm always forgetting what I'm working on in therapy. I'm still sleeping about eighteen hours a day, but it's never enough. I constantly feel like a decrepit ninety year old, not a sparky ninety year old.

My brain still feels like it's going to explode through my skull. The massive ten inch icicle continues to be constantly shoved through my left inner eye socket and into my brain. Just recently, I've developed a technique to somewhat deal with the pain. I brace my left elbow, against my knee or a table, and push the tip of my thumb, as hard as I can, into my inside eye socket. Unfortunately, the relief lasts only as long as I intensely press.

Inside and outside, I'm wearing earplugs and sunglasses, but they don't solve the problem. I'm always covering my eyes and squinting to avoid any light – a 25 watt light bulb is way too bright. When the radio or T.V. is turned on, I quickly cover my ears. The pain from any light and sound is excruciating.

I've had to give up my vocation, all social activities, and my driver's license. I'm also no longer in charge of my money, decisions are made *for* me, and I've lost 95% of my friends. Since the accident, I've moved three times. For now, I'm an inpatient at rehab, but after I'm discharged, I don't know where I'm going to live. All the humiliating losses have piled up faster than I can name.

Every professional has completed their report, and I'm asked what I think. It takes me forever to say, I thought you liked me, but my words are as broken as my spirit. There's a collective "Ohhh." Someone speaks up, "Cathy, we do like you, but we have to tell you the truth."

The meeting ends and everyone goes about their business. In the foreign outside world, people are moving forward and living life. While I remain imprisoned in my brain, craving what is seemingly beyond reach – I need to be the person I used to be. I need my life back. I need to be normal again. I look in the mirror; my face is the image of someone who's IQ is below 70. I feel like a non-entity and consider suicide, but I don't have the courage or energy to do it.

A powerful passion rises within me which helps to change my mind-set. Frig this label and diagnosis, this is not the real me! This is not who I am inside my brain! Even though everyone else believes there's no hope of complete recovery from the TBI, I have to have hope. I decide to continue working diligently at rehab, and to continue delving deeper into my precious inner awareness training. One day, I will be completely liberated from this TBI, and I will be reconnected – *no matter what anyone else says.*

THE GRUELING ROAD OF RECOVERY

I'm working tenaciously at rehab. The doctors and therapists are very happy with my minute improvements. Not me. I am light years away from where I was pre-TBI. I keep asking for more therapies because I need to completely recover as quickly as I can, and thankfully I receive them. With every test result and doctor's appointment at rehab and Beth Israel, I'm constantly bombarded with an endless list of "No's and Never's" and "Impossible's"

"You will never be able to do anything physical, ever again." "No, you cannot be in charge of your money." "No, you cannot drive." "No, you cannot garden." "You will never work with wood again." "You have to understand, the brain is a very complex organ, and we're in the infancy of understanding the brain. However, *we know it's impossible to heal the brain!*" "You have to accept what we say – *you will never, ever recover.*" "No, Never..." The barrage of "No's and Never's" is vastly more challenging than the Herculean task of trying to get information, into and out of, the prison in my brain. With each new "No and Never," it feels like I'm being knocked down, again and again.

To square away my mind-set and keep moving forward, I think about what a friend always says: Keep your eye on the ball, and you'll be okay. I decide that, instead of focusing on all *their* negatives and "No's and Never's," I will keep developing my inner awareness, and do the best job I can at rehab.

Next, I focus on my improvements; I've reached a deeper level of inner awareness. I'm now aware of subtle changes of energy between people and in situations; however, I don't know what these energy changes mean. Second, although I'm still not able to follow people's words because they're speaking way too fast. I'm hoping that delving deeper into my inner awareness training will guide me in how to connect what's happening inside my body to understand people's energies and words. Third, deep in my gut, I sense that I need to keep my brain healing journey to myself. I know that if I tell people, especially at rehab, they'll send me for more counseling because I haven't "accepted" the TBI. The last thing I need from the foreign outside world is more obstacles. I take a breath, and set my sights, on delving deeper into my precious inner awareness training, and discovering a way to liberate and reconnect myself.

BETTER ATTITUDE BETTER TREATMENT

I'm sitting in a waiting area for my next therapy appointment at rehab. Since the TBI, I spend a lot of time waiting. I'm distracted by two therapists standing close by having a conversation. They can see me, and I can hear them quite well. I catch a word or two, but they're speaking way too fast for me to understand them. Unintentionally, I become aware of my inner body and how it's responding. My whole torso is open, warm, and relaxed. Next, I'm aware of a vibrant energy coming from deep inside the therapists' bodies and exuding outward. Then, I notice their body language; they are full of life and have genuine smiles on their faces. I connect the clues: first, I always start with my inner awareness training – being aware of how my inner body is responding; second, the therapist's inner energy; and third, their body language. I continue being aware of how my inner body is responding, and I catch a few more words. I realize they're talking about a patient's great attitude and work ethic, but they don't mention his name.

Step by step, I'm discovering that – my inner awareness; how my inner body responds, matches the energy and intent of people and situations. My ability to understand the foreign outside world and how it works continues to improve – as long as I'm focusing on delving deeper into my inner awareness training. Otherwise, I don't have a clue as to what's happening in the foreign outside world. The key to my brain healing journey continues to be my precious inner awareness training.

One therapist looks directly at and through me; then, looks in the opposite direction, down the hall. I sense that she's making sure no one is listening. How could she not see me, I'm right near them? She leans toward the other therapist and talks about how much she admires the patient; his attitude and desire to get better. Proudly she states, "I try to give him extra help when I can."

My inner body becomes cold and closed. Inside, I'm aware the energy of both therapists has completely changed – negative gunk is oozing from inside their closed bodies then outward. *My inner awareness is spot on*; their voices are tense as they talk about a very negative patient. They're sharing that he's always miserable and complains about everything. They're also discussing how difficult it is to deal with negative people. I sense one therapist is getting quite frustrated. A few seconds later she blurts out. "I don't like to say it, but I can't wait for his session to be over." The other therapist coldly states, "He's given up. You've got to accept it." Their conversation ends, and they return to work. Being invisible has its advantages. Unknowingly, they've helped me to delve deeper into my inner awareness training. Thankfully, this will be the only time that I hear therapists talking about patients at rehab.

People in the foreign outside world think nothing much is happening inside my being. They don't have a clue. *When I focus on delving deeper into my inner awareness training; I'm able to connect how my inner body is responding to the interactions of people and situations in the foreign outside world. Inside, I'm able to make decisions and plan, ask and answer questions, focus on finding positive, healthy solutions, reflect, and much more. Unfortunately, the thick, blurry glass wall prevents the vast majority of words and information from passing through this massive barrier, in either direction.*

Inside the prison in my brain, I contemplate the therapists' conversation, and other people's conversations. I've learned that people with good attitudes and work ethic, and who are friendly and courteous receive better treatment. Fortunately, before the accident, I had worked at having a great attitude and interpersonal skills. Taking everything into account, I make a plan. I decide to be a "good patient" and to get to know the staff a little better. Before each therapy, I try to remember to ask the therapist about their day, or if they had a good weekend. If they're into sports, I ask about the big game. I'll keep things light and friendly because I don't want to be like the "icky, creepy patient."

In the beginning, each therapist plays the "professional card," responding politely when I ask about their day. Over time, some professionals seem more open and comfortable, I believe it's because they sense my sincerity. Slowly, I get to know some of the professionals, and I experience our common human-ness; they're regular people. I sense genuine compassion exuding from deep within them; they truly want to help people.

Another therapy session is ending and the therapist is reminding me of my next appointment. I'm having a tough time listening, because I'm trying to remember to thank her for all her help. Before I leave the room, I thank her. Deep inside, I know it's important to thank people, especially those who've been very kind. My hope is that after I've completely liberated myself from this prison in my brain and have been reconnected, I'll have the opportunity to properly thank all of them for their extraordinary care and kindness.

This is a good time to reflect on my brain healing journey. It's colder, the leaves are off the trees, and people are wearing coats. Thankfully, my brain no longer feels like its going to explode out my skull. The professionals at rehab continue to be delighted with my minuscule progress. I'm not. I want to be improving by leaps and bounds, but I'm still light years away from where I was pre-TBI. *Every* therapy and task in the foreign outside world feels like I'm trying to summit Mt. Everest, during a blizzard, without oxygen. Although therapy at rehab is grueling and frustrating, if you combine all of the therapies, they don't even come close to the confounding speech therapy. I diligently try to speak, but

I still don't know where the words are in my brain. I also still sound like a little, little kid. But, little kids learn to speak. Will I?

On the plus side, when I'm aware of how my inner body is responding while doing a task in therapy etc. – there is a small improvement in my ability to focus on the task. But, when I'm not aware of my inner body, I completely flounder.

I wonder, why am I making such great progress with my inner awareness training and why is it so easy to do? Yet my brain is still completely useless. Is my inner awareness improving because there isn't an option of relying on my brain? Hmm, if I had an intact brain, would it be this simple and natural to develop my inner awareness? I believe so. On the other hand, if I didn't have a busted brain, I probably wouldn't have put in the small amount of time and effort to develop this phenomenal inner skill. I would have *solely* relied on my brain to understand people and situations which means; I would have gone through life with a handicap. Now that's hilarious! My sense of humor is gradually awakening and helping me to keep on keeping on.

HUMOR AND
SONG
NO PC HERE

I can laugh or cry about the TBI and my life. Although I've done my share of crying, laughter keeps my spirit strong. Since entering rehab, many of my friends have disappeared. Fortunately, other patients have become my new friends. We self-identify as gimps and no-brainers – our gallows humor helps keep our spirit up. We tell the sickest stories and laugh about our lives. The amputees tell great jokes. Unfortunately, I'm not able to remember them. They also share about their recoveries and enormous challenges. Inside, it's easy for me to sense their pain of losing a limb, dealing with prosthesis, and families and friends. Though the road they're traveling is filled with obstacles, they have a positive attitude; nothing is going to stop them. They inspire me to keep persevering forward, *no matter what.*

One of my amputee buddies jokingly says, "Yea, it's a tough road to hoe." Everyone laughs. I start telling a TBI joke, but I can't remember the joke or the punch line. A gimp friend smiles and says. "Now, that's a no-brainer joke!" We laugh and laugh. I'm laughing so hard, tears are flowing down my face, and I'm having a hard time catching my breath. It feels good to be laughing again.

My favorite song since the TBI is "If I only had a brain…," from the Wizard of Oz, I think of it as my no-brainer national anthem. I smile from ear to ear and sing with gusto, "If I only had a brain," then hum the rest of song because I've forgotten the words. Some people have a really hard time that I use gallows humor to deal with the TBI and all the losses. I don't let them stop me. I smile and make sure to sing and hum even louder my national anthem when I'm around people who think I'm not politically correct. I will not allow people or anything to get in the way; I will do whatever it takes to succeed in my brain healing journey. Joking about my self and the TBI is a great tool that helps stoke the fire in my belly – persevere forward. I figure if laughing about myself and the TBI, and using gallows humor to deal with my situation helps so be it. I'm not going to let some friggin busted brain beat me.

PERSEVERING - -
IT'S A
DIRECTIONAL
THING

People are wearing big, thick coats and it's really cold outside; winter is my least favorite time of year. Not only is it bleak outside, all my no-brainer friends and the next set have disappeared. Although people begin their recovery process on different days and weeks at the rehabilitation hospital, I notice about every season, there's a new bunch of no-brainers, and I don't know why. In a hallway, I ask a therapist where my friend's are. Fortunately, she understands my broken speech. She takes a deep, long breath, and while she's exhaling, I sense a shift occurring within her. She's totally discouraged. Wow, I have never been aware, then seen her, or any rehab professional down; they're usually so upbeat.

Eventually she says, "They're no longer coming to rehab." I am shocked. I miss my friends. I also don't want to go down the same road they did. *I need to completely heal my brain and be reconnected.* I keep asking her, why aren't my friends coming to rehab? Inside, I sense another change in her energy; then, I notice her body language. She's not closed; it's more like she's not sure how to answer. I can tell she's hesitating, hoping I'll forget. But, it's my inner body that has the question and needs an answer, not my busted brain. I love my inner awareness training and that, step by step, it's helping me understand the foreign outside world. Finally, she accepts that I'm not going away and speaks the truth no one wants to admit. "Many people are not willing to do all the work. Before they complete their therapy, they stop coming to rehab."

I am stunned. The thought of *not* doing rehab hasn't crossed my mind. Giving up is *not* an option. *I am desperate; I will do anything to recover. I've got to completely heal my brain! I've got to be reconnected!* I look at the therapist; her body is open, and her heart is filled with sadness and compassion. Everything matches; she's being truthful. The rehab staff doesn't want their patients giving up; they're rooting for us to succeed. But, the responsibility to do all the work, to get all the results, rests squarely on each patient's shoulders.

This experience profoundly affects me. Instead of focusing on the negatives, I decide to research why some people diligently persevere forwards while others give up or persevere backwards. My research will take place where I spend the vast majority of time, at rehab. I try to schedule my rides, the short bus, to arrive earlier to rehab in order to talk with and observe as many people as possible; people with brain problems, other patients, and their families and friends. Life is interesting, as a kid I'd laugh uncomfortably when others made fun of the "short bus" and the kids with problems in it. Now, I'm riding the short bus, and I'm grateful for the rides to and from rehab.

I approach a waiting area and see Jeff; he has a TBI, sitting with his parents. Slowly, I ask how they're all doing. His parents tell me fine, but Jeff says nothing. Jeff's head is hung low, and his eyes are glued to the floor. Jeff's energy is all closed up – his energy reminds me of someone who's given up.

Though I see Jeff on a regular basis, for the first time I ask him how it's going at rehab. In a weak voice, he talks about how people keep telling him everything he can't do and won't ever be able to do. He doesn't want to do this therapy or any therapy. His life sucks, and he'll never be ok, so why try. Why try? With each word his voice trails off to barely a whisper while his give-up energy grows stronger.

His mom cheerfully says, "You've got to keep trying. You can't give-up." His dad chimes in, "C'mon buddy, you can do this. You can do this!" In my broken speech, I slowly share how difficult it is to have a TBI, thankfully, they understand me. Here's the gist of what I very slowly say, 'So many times, I've wanted to give-up, especially after receiving another heartbreaking "No and Never" and "Impossible." It's utterly frustrating, not being able to do the simple, easy things I did as a kid. But, I've got to keep trying, and focus on the positives – what's working and how much I've improved. *I know, one day I'll be able to do everything I did before and do them better. I've got to always have hope, and to always keep trying, no matter what.'*

Despite our encouragement, Jeff's entrenched in utter hopelessness. A therapist pops her head out the door and enthusiastically asks Jeff if he's ready. He lets out a long, discouraging sigh. Without raising his head, he slowly walks into the physical therapy room.

A few moments later, his parents share how it's a fight to get him to come to rehab and do the work at home. They wish he had a better attitude, but he's given up. They wish they could do his therapies for him, but they know they can't. My heart aches; it's easy to sense how much they love and want to help Jeff. They just want their son back. In time I'll realize that in some ways, families and friends have it harder emotionally, because they're not able to do the therapies, etc. for their loved one. Though they love, support, and encourage their loved one, many feel it's not enough. Jeff's parents spark up. They ask how I persevere and have a great attitude. It's easy to sense; they're hoping to hear a magic solution.

Here's the gist of what I very slowly say in my broken speech, 'TBI sucks, and I'm grieving massive losses, including not being able to do all the things I did before the TBI. But, it's no excuse for having a bad attitude. For me to get my life back; it's crucial that I decide to be positive, to *always* focus on and feed myself: listen, read, and watch things that inspire me, consistently take positive actions, and to choose to hang out with people who are positive. Also to always, always, ALWAYS have hope, *no matter what*. I've learned that it's much easier and less work to be positive than negative. I wasn't born with a good attitude and persevering forwards, and people aren't born with a bad attitude and giving up. In fact, years ago, I worked my butt off to turn around my bad attitude into a positive, healthy one. That's a story for another day.

Every person makes a decision about how they: think, speak, act, and live. No one can change another. The responsibility for your son's attitude rests squarely on his shoulders. Don't let his negative attitude get to you. Keep having a positive attitude, encourage, and love him. That's all you can do.'

Silence. While I was trying to get the words out, I sensed they already knew what to do – people do, sometimes they just need a reminder. After a long, pregnant pause, they tell me that they understand, but they wish they could do more. Before the season ends, Jeff and his parents are no longer coming to rehab.

I also do my research in the open rooms of physical and occupational therapy. Diagonally across from me, at another table, is a big, burly man who seems as though he was very intelligent before his brain problem. Day after day, he battles through frustrations and tears trying to do second grade math problems. In the middle of a session, I'm startled by his booming, broken voice: "I did it!" His fists are pumping in the air. Inside, it's easy to sense the pride exuding from him. The big, burly man motivates me to keep on persevering, especially when I don't want to.

On the opposite end of the spectrum, it's difficult to watch grown adults throw things, cry, stop working, and sit back in their chair absolutely dejected. It's easy to sense then see their overwhelming frustration. They *too* don't understand basic instructions and are unable to do the simplest tasks. Though each therapist encourages them to keep trying, they've totally given up. More than a few people have stormed out in the middle of therapy, vowing never to come back, and they don't.

In addition to all my therapies, I'm also attending different groups at rehab. In one group, a woman with her body all puffed up like a peacock is cheerfully announcing, over and over again. "I've got brain damage. I can't do anything. I've got all these limitations. I've got to accept what the doctors say. I've got brain damage…" At first, I think she's nuts and start writing her off. *Until I realize that what's happening inside my body is not matching her energy and words. I'm experiencing a new level of inner awareness.* Although her words sound upbeat, my body is closed to protect itself from the onslaught of her negative energy which is irritating and repelling me like a magnet.

I continue paying attention to my inner body while she keeps repeating her mantra. Her energy reminds me of being proud, but it's not the same kind of pride as that of the big, burly man. With his pride, my body was open, relaxed, and I felt energized. Her pride is draining and depressing. I understand that part of what's happening is a result of her brain problems; however, I sense the energy exuding from her is a different kind of give-up energy.

Everything becomes clear when she explains, in a roundabout way, that she didn't know who she was pre-TBI. Now that she has a TBI, she has an identity. I am shocked. She's wearing the TBI like a badge of honor. In time, other people with brain problems will disclose that they now have an identity because of the TBI or other brain problems. My gut is letting me know that *– the last thing I need to do is accept the TBI. Frig that. If I accept the TBI, I will die imprisoned in my brain, and there's no way I'm going to let that happen.*

In a different group, we play board games. A bunch of no-brainers playing board games is not a pretty sight. We're constantly forgetting what game we're playing, whose turn it is, and whose color piece is whose. I feel for the occupational therapist; her job reminds me of trying to herd a bunch of slow cats moving in all different directions. At times, we get frustrated and grumble a bit, but we keep trying. Before the TBI, I liked playing board games and other games. Now, I detest playing games. However, if playing board games or other games will help free me from this prison in my brain, I'm all in.

In another group, there are two vastly different versions of people persevering. One guy, with a TBI, complains about everything and vehemently refuses to try. He gives all sorts of excuses: the work is too hard, he doesn't want to struggle, and he wants everything easy, like it was before. Yet, he has an abundance of energy to blame, complain, make excuses, and he is diligently working at getting others to give-up. I get a bad sense from him. My inner body is closed and cold when I'm around him. His energy reminds me of putting up both hands to stop; it's like he's fortifying his massive, self-imposed prison of negativity. The therapist and some of us no-brainers encourage him. But, he says it's too hard to change his attitude or try. A few of us no-brainers look at each other and shake our heads. I can sense and smell his BS. Again, the therapist encourages him to try, but he won't listen. In the same group, there's a woman who is a mountain of strength. She can only see one side of a computer screen or piece of paper. But, she works diligently, trying to see the whole screen and paper. The energy exuding from her is pure determination. She inspires me to succeed at what people say is impossible.

On another day, I'm in a waiting area, when a new guy with a TBI walks up and sits beside me. Before I can say "hi," he slowly starts listing all his "No's and Never's" and "Impossible's," and that nothing will ever work, so why even try. He tells me that he should just go home, to the house he's lived in for years. He wants to look at the pictures, from the recent vacation he took with his family. Next, he tells me – I should give-up, too.

My back is rising up big time. Before I speak, I calm down somewhat. Even so, I'm rather blunt; here's the gist of what I say in my very slow broken speech. 'Dude! You and I are facing the same thing, except you still have your home, and you went on vacation. I don't have any of that. Yet, *I still have a positive attitude, and I'm working my butt off to get better. You and every other person can have a positive attitude and do all the work to get all the results, no matter what the heck is going on in life, including TBI. Dude, I'm not giving up, so don't even go there.'*

Inside, I sense I need to be more compassionate. I take a breath before I speak, 'Man, there are times I don't want to do the work or have a good attitude, especially after hearing another "No and Never." Just like you, and everyone else with brain problems, I've experienced massive loss, and I'm grieving. But, I've already decided that I'm not going to turn around, go backwards, and barely exist in negativity land. Be honest; there are no doctors or therapists here. You want the results, but you don't want to do the work. You're looking for a magic wand or pill.' He gives me a slick smile; he's been caught in his BS. Rather than change his mindset, he decides to take the harder route, he continues diligently blaming, complaining, and making all kinds of excuses. I wonder how much progress he'd make if he'd put his energy into doing the work and having a positive attitude; it certainly be a much easier and enjoyable way to live. A few minutes later, he abruptly stands up. He is absolutely infuriated that I won't agree with him, that I won't have a bad attitude, and that I won't give-up. As he walks away, I have no idea that this is the last time I'll see him.

I remember an event that happened years before the TBI. I was having a wonderful conversation with an old timer; he was in his seventies, and I was in my mid 20's. A man walked up and interrupted us. He told us everything that was wrong in his life and everyone who was responsible for *all* his problems. His list was endless: job, relationship, kids, mortgage, not having a boat, and so on. The man was in mid-breath when the old timer shared a sentiment I'd heard many times from other friends and mentors. "If everything around you stinks, it's time to take a bath." The man was surprised and asked the old timer what he meant. The old timer calmly said, "There's only one thing you can change, that's the person you see in the mirror. Take a look at yourself, rather than blame others. When you shift your attitude, by being grateful and taking full responsibility for your thinking, words, actions, and life, you'll experience something every person wants – peace of mind. Even if everything outside of you stays the same, you can have something no one can give you, and no one can take away – a happiness that comes from deep inside." The man stood there with his mouth open. A few seconds later, the man turned and walked away without saying a word. I don't know if he ever understood those profound, simple words of wisdom. I did and still do.

For many years, I've known that every human being is an expert at persevering. People are constantly making decisions and taking actions that move them forwards or backwards. There's no such thing as staying the same or moving only in one direction. The same process is used to persevere forwards or backwards – the difference is the direction. To persevere forwards a healthy decision is made, consistent positive actions are taken, people learn from their successes and missteps, and repeat. The best time to make the decision to persevere forwards is right now. Persevering forwards is not picking your self up by the bootstraps and it certainly isn't being a cockeyed optimist. To persevere backwards or give up, an unhealthy decision is made, consistent negative actions are taken, people don't learn from their successes and missteps, and repeat. Giving up might seem like the easier option at times, but the damage it does destroying the spirit is too high of a price to pay.

Each person works diligently in their pursuit to be as happy or as miserable as they choose, and it only takes a moment to change direction. It's simple, moment by moment, every person makes a decision about how they: think, speak, act, and live, and the responsibility to change and grow, or wither rests squarely on each person's shoulders. Whether people choose to be responsible is another topic.

Years ago, I transformed negative thinking into positive, and persevering backwards into moving forwards. In my experience, (which I'll share throughout the book) it is immensely easier to have a positive attitude, persevere forwards, be passionate about what I'm doing, and be grateful for even the smallest things – no matter what. How do I continue improving? I'm very conscious of what I input into my life and who I hang out with.

I think of a positive attitude, persevering forward, being passionate, and grateful like I think of food. Eating one meal will not fill me for the rest of my life. Every day, and throughout the day, I need to purposefully feed my mind with things that encourage and give me hope, and to be around people who inspire me to be the best person I can be. Just as important, I need to intentionally close my mind to all negatives. In life I've faced big and small challenges, just like everyone else. The tough times are a little easier and pass a little more quickly, and the great times are more enjoyable and last longer by having a positive attitude, persevering forward, being passionate, and grateful.

In every cell of my being, I know the TBI is just a temporary situation, despite every professional's diagnosis. I've made a conscious decision not to accept or own the TBI. I know if I accepted the TBI, my thinking would turn around, and next thing I know, I'd be heading backwards. I'm not in denial that I have a TBI; this is all about self-preservation. I refuse to exist in the thick, blurry glass wall for the rest of my life, only to die imprisoned in my brain. How long will it take to be free, I don't know. What I do know is that it's not a question of if; my mind-set is when I'm free and reconnected.

The power that drives my brain healing journey is pretty simple; a mammoth desire from deep inside to be completely liberated from the prison in my brain, in order to be fully reconnected; to be home within me – my body, then with everyone and everything. I will do whatever it takes to get me back.

I've learned a few things from my research, most I already know. From the negative people, they've reinforced what I already know. Don't follow in their footsteps; basically, don't do what doesn't work. It's disheartening to watch people's lives spiral down the toilet, especially when they keep reaching up to flush. Their enormous determination to give-up or persevere backwards is astounding. Some people seem to take pleasure in their misery, and it gets old listening to them focus on everything that's wrong and what they can't do. They also talk on and on and on about "*my* TBI, *my* stroke, *my* _____(fill in the blank). You won't hear me say that; it's the TBI or TBI; again, I do not own or accept the TBI. In addition, a few people have said that

I'm able to persevere and they can't. BULL! That's just another ridiculous excuse. Having a TBI, or dealing with other tough things in life isn't an excuse for having a weak ass mind-set and not doing all the work. I wonder, would people do all the work if they didn't believe the negativity of the "No's and Never's" and "Impossible's?" Would they do all the work if there was a way to completely heal the brain? Would they have a different attitude? Or, would they continue vigorously feeding their negativity? I don't know.

There's no room in my journey for the enormous heavy weight and draining energy of negativity, persevering backwards, give-up, slackers, naysayers, haters, gossipers, doubts, etc. This self-defeating mind-set will only take me off course. I decide to stop getting to know or sit near the "want to, want to's" with their give-up energy – people who want the results, but they won't do all the work to get the results. I know the negative people will not last, and I will not be pulled under by the drain of their wake. I accept people's decision and watch them leave the rehabilitation hospital long before they leave the building.

From the positive people, I've learned to put aside my pride, to not focus on who I used to be, nor what I think I should be able to do right now. They've helped me to reinforce that I need to keep focusing on the task at hand, on what works, and how much I've improved.

To my surprise there are other benefits from my research. First, my inner awareness has grown by leaps and bounds; it's so simple and getting easier and easier to delve deeper into my training. I no longer have to consciously focus on being aware of my inner body; it's natural. Second, being and staying aware of my inner body has improved my focus on tasks in the foreign outside world and energy level a tiny, tiny bit. On the other hand, when I'm not aware of my inner body; I completely flounder.

While doing my research I had a surprising insight. People have been very open; they shared with me differently than how they talked with the professionals. I believe they were comfortable because I'm one of them, and I'm honored and grateful for their trust.

Though I've improved a bit from the *inside out*, the thick, blurry glass prison is completely intact. I'm also still completely disconnected from everyone and everything in the foreign outside world, including my body. Again, I consciously decide not to focus on these facts. Having a positive attitude and persevering forward doesn't mean I ignore the fact that I have a TBI or the other tough things I've faced in life. Once more, I consciously choose to continue focusing on the *easier and more enjoyable path*; having a positive mind-set, persevering forward, being passionate, and grateful. Am I perfect at being positive and persevering forwards? No. No one is perfect. However, I do give my absolute best; to the best of my ability.

Again, I make a conscious decision to completely liberate myself from the prison in my brain, to be fully reconnected, and to enjoy each step in my brain healing journey. How do I do this? Once again, I make a healthy decision, consistently take positive actions, learn and grow from my successes and missteps, and repeat – *no matter what*.

3

SERVICE IS OUR HIGHEST CALLING

It is refreshing to be in the presence of people who look me *in* the eye, talk *with* me as a fellow human being, and most importantly, their energy matches their words and actions. In my broken speech, I often thank them for their kindness. After I've completely liberated myself from the TBI and I'm reconnected, I look forward to effortlessly expressing my profound gratitude to them. Here are a few stories of people whose strength and acts of humanity inspire me to always strive to be a better human being.

DAD - PMA KID
POSITIVE
MENTAL
ATTITUDE

Dad is the only person who knew me before the TBI and interacts with me daily, who still treats me as an adult. It's most heartening that he speaks with me, not down or around me. Since the TBI, Dad has stepped up big time. He is extraordinarily patient, calm, and exudes compassion which is totally out of character. Normally, he is gruff, impatient, and definitely not a touchy-feely type of person. Dad and I have developed as close of a relationship as is possible, considering the thick, blurry glass prison in my brain. He has a standing order when I call him at work; I'm to be put through, no matter what, even if he's with the president of the company. What's interesting is that before the accident, Dad and I weren't close, at all. In fact, the best way to describe my biological family is screwed up, but that's a story for later on.

Dad's developed fun, simple, and ingenious ways to stimulate my brain. He encourages me to count simple numbers, whether on the license plate in front of us at stoplights or playing cribbage. I'm grateful that he lets me use my fingers to count because at rehab they won't. Unfortunately, no matter how much I try, I don't know what numbers are and how to add them.

Finally, he tells me 4 + 5 = 9. I keep trying and trying to get into my brain that 4 + 5 = 9, but it just won't go in.

When I get frustrated or down, whether it's counting numbers, trying to get the words out, or anything else, he'll use his favorite saying: PMA, Kid! Positive Mental Attitude! I think he'll always call me kid; it's his way of showing that he cares and loves me. Also, his upbeat voice as he says, "PMA, Kid" and his energy helps turn around my attitude. I treasure all his support; it's positively affecting my brain healing journey. My hope is that more people deal with each other as Dad treats me – as a fellow human being.

THE FIRST TBI SURVIVORS GROUP IN THE COUNTRY

Dad and I are in the hallway of the Brain Injury Unit at rehab. I'm trying to talk, and as usual, the words aren't coming out right. My body is tense, and I'm getting frustrated. Gently, Dad says, "Calm down. It's not going to help you get the word by being frustrated. Relax, calm down."

Maybe it's his tone, his timing, or his simple words. For whatever reason, I calm down and feel better. Though I'm still not able to get the words out, my very short attention span finally becomes an asset. I'm distracted by a flyer on the bulletin board, but I'm unable to read it. Dad reads the flyer, and tells me there's a Survivor Group for People with Brain Injuries; it's the first group in the country. Enthusiastically, he asks if I want to go. There's a spark in his eyes and they're misty. There's also something else I haven't seen in a long time – hope. I nod my head up and down. Dad smiles, I think he's more excited than I am.

As usual, I completely forget about the meeting. A few days later, after supper, Dad tells me it's time to go. I have no idea where we're going, I'm just happy to be with my Dad. We get in the car, and he reminds me about the Survivor Group meeting for People with Brain Injuries. *My head drops; I do not want to go to that meeting with those people. I don't want to admit to myself, or anyone else, that I really do have a TBI. It's not a denial thing. I believe that it's positive not to accept the TBI.* I'm aware that my body is tight and I'm stressing big time about the meeting. Calmly, Dad asks if I want him to go to the meeting. I look up, and nod my head up and down. I am so relieved.

The meeting is at a local library in Burlington, MA. We enter the library, go downstairs, and I peek through the small rectangular glass window with wire mesh in the door. The room is filled with people. Dad and I sit behind a woman with a huge German Shepherd dog. After a few minutes, I become aware that the woman is blind. Then, I smell the worst, raunchy, putrid odor I've *ever* smelled, and it's coming from her dog. My eyes are watering. I don't know what she feeds her dog, but he has the worst farts ever. I look at Dad; we're both trying not to laugh, which is making us want to laugh even more.

Despite the outrageous smell, it's easy to sense genuine compassion in the room; people are warm, open, and kind. I meet some of the most brilliant people who have a TBI; PhDs, homemakers, academics, medical professionals, and teachers, etc. We all have one thing in common, our minds are like scrambled eggs. TBI does not discriminate; it affects all kinds of people, and it doesn't care about your education level, cultural background, race, sex, finances, or anything else.

People freely share about their lives; it's like they're telling my story. They understand the constant and utter exhaustion, the inability to remember, the overwhelming losses, and how excruciatingly difficult it is to do the simplest task. No one is complaining; they're just being honest. I also really like the gallows humor, it keeps the meeting lively. Now that's really funny, a lively TBI meeting.

DR. PETERSON AND THE PROFESSIONAL STAFF

My inner awareness training continues to improve by leaps and bounds, which is helping me to better understand people and situations in the foreign outside world. It's easy to sense the energy of mutual respect and kindness between my team of doctors, nurses, and therapy specialists of all kinds. Again, this is more than a profession; they genuinely care and give their very best.

In between therapy appointments, I see one of my therapists, a naturally compassionate person, talking with her new supervisor. The boss's energy is not very nice, and though she's smiling, it's fake. It's easy to sense the change of energy with the therapist; she is containing her generous, kind nature. The boss walks away and with each step, the therapist's natural compassionate energy and smile returns. I love my inner awareness training; it's making my brain healing journey so much easier and fun!

At each therapy session, I'm always asked, "How are you? What's going on?" I'm from New England; I'm self-reliant and like taking care of any situation. But, since the TBI, I don't have an off-switch in my brain. I feel like the TV character Sophia on the Golden Girls. She had a stroke and says whatever is on her mind. But, I'm not sharp and quick like her. In my broken speech, I'll barely mention something getting in the way: a scheduling problem, a family situation, etc. Within a few days, the problem is magically resolved, and I have no clue how it happened.

Until one day, I ask a question. I finally feel confident to trust Dr. Peterson with something that happened shortly after the TBI. In my broken speech, I ask if gay people become straight after a TBI. She is stunned! Inside, I sense great concern. She asks, "What brings this on?" I try to explain that the neurologists at Beth Israel told me this happens. Her answer is definite and succinct. "No. That is not true." I leave the appointment, and of course, forget about our conversation. A few days later, a rehab neuro-psychologist pulls me aside. She talks with me about getting a new neurologist at Beth Israel. I look at her and wonder, what is she talking about? Then, it's like dawn light on Marblehead. Dr. Peterson is the person responsible for fixing this and so many other challenges. I am grateful for this compassionate leader, doctor, and human being, her positive influence extends throughout the entire hospital.

THE NON-MEDICAL STAFF AT REHAB

Throughout rehab, there's an atmosphere of respect, kindness, and understanding. I'm not a patient, or Cathy the Patient. I'm Cathy, a fellow human being who needs help. The thoughtful, gentleness exuding from the staff is inspiring and comforting.

Since the TBI, I always forget to eat. When I'm having even more difficulty in a therapy session, which is hard to imagine, the smart therapist asks if I've eaten. I shrug my shoulders. Their question becomes more precise. "Are you hungry?" I think for a long, long time. Finally, I say, "Think so."

I'm sent to the cafeteria, where I see Rosita. Even though lunch is almost over, she patiently helps me, once again. I try to tell her how much I appreciate her kindness and how blessed I am to have her as a friend. Though my words are messed up, I can tell she understands by the warmth and kindness exuding from her.

My perspective about life has changed since the TBI. Life is not about things, jobs, money, how busy a person is, or what a person does. Life is about connecting and relating with people, and being of service. Extraordinary human beings come in all sizes, shapes, and do all sorts of work.

KINDNESS AND SUPPORT IN THE MOST UNLIKELY PLACE

Dad and I are off to rehab, but he seems really anxious. He hasn't told me that he needs to set up a payment plan in order for me to continue going to rehab. We enter rehab and I sense his anxiety level rising big time; it's like he's on a mission. Before he crosses the threshold of the business office, he takes a deep breath and exhales.

He talks with the receptionist, and we're sent to a woman whose desk is sort of in the middle of this large room. As we're approaching her, she stands up and shakes our hands. Inside, it's very easy to sense her warmth, kindness, and great desire to help. She's a nice woman. I'm not able to follow their conversation. Although inside I can tell it's going well; Dad has calmed down big time. Throughout the conversation, Dad and the nice woman look over and smile at me. Compassionate energy is going back and forth between them and toward me. I love my inner awareness training.

They finish talking and smile at me; I sense they're delighted. Although I don't have a clue as to what just happened, they've set up a payment plan; I can continue going to all my therapies at rehab. I get a strong gut sense that I'm supposed to say something, but I don't know what to do. I look at Dad, he just keeps smiling. In a little kid voice, I ask Dad if what just happened is good. His smile widens. Exuding from him is relief and gratitude as he says, "Yes, it is very good." There's a palpable feeling of kindness and gratitude filling me and surrounding the three of us. Inwardly, I'm aware that this woman has helped me enormously, but it's my inner body that 100% knows this, not my busted brain. Dad says our business is done and it's time to go. He shakes the nice business woman's hand and thanks her. I shake her hand while smiling and nodding my head up and down. As we're leaving, I look back. The nice business woman is still standing, with her big smile and gentle open heart.

I continue working diligently at rehab, and of course completely forget what happened in the business office. One day, I'm downstairs, on my way to speech therapy when I see a woman halfway down the hall. She's looking directly at me and walking towards me. Instantly, I'm aware that she's been very nice to me. But, I don't know who she is or what she's done. I slow my pace then stop, look to my left and down. I'm desperately trying to remember who she is and what wonderful thing she's done. I gaze up. The nice woman is standing in front of me; her body is open and filled with love. Exuding from her smiling face and body is compassion as she patiently waits. I keep looking to my left and down, then up at her. My mind is blank.

By habit, I put my hands in my jean pockets and touch a piece of paper. The beginning of a memory, slowly, very slowly trickles through the sieve in my brain. It feels like an eternity for a connection to be made. Finally, something connects. She's the nice business woman! I am so excited to hand her the paper that Dad asked me to give her. I don't understand that the paper is a check / money for me to go to rehab. Month after month, the same scenario takes place, with the check Dad gave me, for the nice business woman. The woman's kindness, patience, and understanding are beyond extraordinary.

IT'S A PRESENT
TO BE SEEN

My sister Arlene is three years older, and since the TBI, our relationship has dramatically changed. She's become more like my mom than my sister. Inside, I sense a great deal of compassion and kindness coming from Arlene, as well as grief. *No one* is left untouched by the devastation of brain damage; it's a heavy burden for all.

Arlene is very busy with her two young kids, but she helps me whenever she can, and I appreciate everything she does. Today, we're off to yet another doctor's appointment at Beth Israel. I get in the car, and Arlene asks, "Have you eaten lunch?" *I think and think and think. I can't remember.* She simplifies the question, and slowly asks, "Are you hungry?" *Again, I think for a long time.* Finally I say, "Think so." She smiles, and gently says, "We'll stop and get you something to eat."

Before she puts the car in gear, she reminds me to put on my seatbelt. As I'm putting on my seatbelt, I notice the kids in the back and say, "Hi." In my broken speech, I say to Arlene. "Wow, kids quiet." She laughs, then lowers her voice. "I told them that Aunt Cathy's head hurts a lot, and they need to be really, really quiet and good." I'm shocked and tell her, "Works well." Arlene smiles and says, "Yes, it works very well!"

After my doctor's appointment, we stop at a drugstore. Arlene's walking through the aisles, and I'm following her, just like the kids. We're like a bunch of ducklings following their mother duck, and I'm the duckling that always gets distracted.

A brightly colored kid's toy grabs my attention and after a bit, I look up. I don't see Arlene or the kids; however, I do see a family coming towards me. The older kid is like me, but I think she was born with brain problems. I look at her, and she looks at me. She's speaking all these unspoken words – it's like she's telling me that – she sees me – *inside* the prison in my brain. Wow, I'm taken aback; she really sees me! For the first time since the TBI, someone sees me *inside* the thick, blurry glass wall! Her language is clear. She sees me, but she isn't using words! Why is this kid able to communicate with me, but I'm not able to speak with her? Why isn't anyone from the foreign outside world able to converse with me, inside the prison in my brain? Why don't I know this kid's language? Is this my language? If so, how do I learn this language?

She walks past me and the communication stops. Though this one way contact lasts only a few seconds, I am so very grateful for the gift of being seen. *Another human being really saw me, inside the prison in my brain! She saw ME!* I want to dance in the aisle, but I'm not the athletic, surefooted person I once was. At the time, I didn't know this would be the one and only contact inside the thick, blurry glass wall in my brain.

I wonder: is having a TBI the same or similar to people born with brain problems? Do they have a thick, blurry glass prison in their brain? Are they like me, disconnected and unable to break out of their prison? Do they know there's a foreign outside world? Do they want to be connected with the outside world?

A pre-TBI memory floats across my mind. I contemplate what people have said, and what I've said about people with brain problems. "He's locked within his own world. I wish, I knew how to get through to him." "I know she's in there, but I'm not able to connect with her. I wonder, what it's like inside her world." "I wish I could reach in and grab him back."

Life is funny. Before the TBI, I was on the outside trying to look into *their* world. I believed people with brain problems were slow, unintelligent, and there wasn't much going on inside their minds. I couldn't have been more wrong. Now, I'm imprisoned in my brain and desperately trying to find a way out. No one, including me talks about the thick, blurry glass wall, or their version of the prison in their brain? Am I the only one having this experience? Are we all so imprisoned that we're unable to talk about the thick, blurry glass wall? I don't know, and I am tired of saying that I don't know. Maybe one day, someone will develop a two-way communication and tests that can penetrate the thick, blurry glass prison wall in the brain. I desperately want to tell people that I am smarter and that there's a heck of a lot more going on inside these prison walls than their test results. But, wishing or waiting for these tests and communication to be developed will not help me now.

I yearn to be free, to be reconnected, and to be home. There has to be a way to navigate the vast expanse between the prison in my brain and the foreign outside world. I swear, after I'm liberated I will *not* take for granted living free and being connected, like I did before the accident. The memory of the kid in the store comes to mind. If she could communicate through the thick, blurry glass wall – that means there's a way to break through the prison in my brain!

4

THE LAST "NO AND NEVER"

The seasons have come full circle. I'm starting to understand, this means it's been about a year since the accident. One year is "the magic number" every professional has said and keeps saying. "Don't expect any more improvement with your brain function after one year." Every time, I'm told about this magic number, I listen and smile appropriately. Inside, I say – Bull!

One by one, each therapist and doctor asks what I want to do with my life. Are they nuts? Who's the one with the busted brain? What about all their "No's and Never's"? Their question gets me thinking about rehab and how effective it is. All my therapies and test results have consistently shown I'm progressing well. Yet, I am still light years away from where I was pre-TBI.

Even though rehab has told me, there's only so much they can do. I have always held out hope, that they would teach me the tools to completely heal my brain – until now. It's obvious, the rehabilitation method does not have a solution to free me from the prison in my brain. I need to find another path. I hear about other no-brainers going to college. Why not me? I figure, making my brain smart *has* to be the way to completely heal my brain because there aren't *any* other options.

Enthusiastically, I try to tell my team that I want to go to college! The energy exuding from their bodies and in the room completely changes. All the therapists and doctors look at each other. They don't say a word, but their energy is speaking volumes. They're all closed up. They don't think I can go to school, and they don't want to tell me. In a roundabout, polite manner, one person speaks up. "It may be too hard for you to go to college."

With all the intensity I can muster, I try to bluntly say that I need to go to school. Again, the looks go from one person to another. They know they're not going to sway me. Finally, a decision is made to do more testing. However, this time the testing will occur at a specialty testing place in Boston. I am so bloody tired of being tested. But, I'll jump through whatever hoops they put in front of me, if it means that I'll be free of this TBI.

For three exhausting days, I'm put through a battery of tests, and I think I've done well. The day arrives for me to get my test results, and I am excited to get the okay to go to school. While waiting for the meeting, I notice a woman walking toward me. She says hello and uses my name, but I don't know her. She tells me that she's my representative from rehab and is here for my meeting. I'm surprised. Why do I need someone from rehab? Although I don't understand, I sense her sincerity and compassionate energy.

Before I can say anything, the professionals who tested me and the rest of their staff walk in, and the meeting begins. The *entire* testing staff turns their back to me. The woman running the meeting politely gives my test results exclusively to the woman from rehab. Once again, I've become the invisible woman, but this time it's different. A huge wall has consciously been built to block me. I look at the woman from rehab; she looks just as stunned as I am. I don't think she knows what to do.

I'm aware that my heart is racing. I take a deep breath, and my exhale comes out quivering. I *need* to stay calm, so I can get the okay to go to school to make my brain smart. Then, I'll be completely healed and reconnected. I want to interrupt, but I have a gut sense not to.

Finally, the testing staff finishes giving their report to the woman from rehab, and they turn towards me. Their energy and the atmosphere of the room totally changes. Icy daggers of hostility are coming from the testing staff and are trying to cut into the core of my being. I shudder. Inside, huge warning signs are going off. Every cell of my being is yelling at me to run or hide behind someone to protect me. The woman running the meeting sets her sights on me. Venomous, menacing energy gunk is welling up inside her body. In a terrorizing, icy cold intimidating voice, she sums up her report in *one sentence.*

"You do NOT have the ability to go to school, and you NEVER will."

Her energy and words stun me. They do not understand. Desperately, I try to explain that I *have* to go to school – going to school is my *last hope* for recovery from the TBI; there are no other options. Nothing I say can pierce their walls. I look for help from the woman from rehab; she is absolutely shocked by their unprofessional callousness. While I'm in mid-sentence, the testing staff stands up and walks away. *Their* meeting is over.

In silence, the woman from rehab and I leave their office. She pushes the elevator button, the door opens, and the deafening roar of *all* the "No's and Never's" and "Impossible's" overpowers me. The door closes, and as we descend, I feel myself falling. I'm utterly disorientated. My tenacious determination has been brutally crushed.

The elevator stops, but I continue falling. Exploding in my brain are the testing staff's agonizing words, and every "No and Never," and "Impossible." "You do NOT have the ability to go to school, and you NEVER will." "You will never, ever recover from TBI." "No, you can't ever do anything physical again." "No, you can't garden." "No, you can't drive." "No, Never, No Never…" I'm being slammed into a state of submission. This is and will be the lowest point of the TBI.

The woman from rehab and I walk across the street to the Boston Common. We stand at the corner, and she asks if I'm depressed. I cannot lift my head. I try to say yes, but I've lost all effort to speak. She says something, but her words are drowned out by every "No and Never" and "Impossible." The woman from rehab leaves.

In utter hopelessness, I descend into the bowels of the "T," the transportation center. I'm overwhelmed by the stench of urine. With each step, the thick, blurry glass prison is shrouded by the deluge of all the "No's and Never's" and "Impossibles." In my mind's eye, the billowy, soft clouds and cool mist has changed into a **forever fall in a never-ending hole of utter darkness**. I've begun to accept my place of entombment in the prison in my brain; my spirit feels like its being severed.

Time passes; it feels like a few days, but I no longer care. I'm hunched over, in the middle of the bedroom. Deep inside I have gut sense. You can get through this, Cathy. You've gone through harder times than TBI. You've not only survived, you've thrived.

5

MY POWERFUL PAST

It's not about how I start my journey. What's important is – this moment – the bearing I set and the consistent actions I take to move forward – right now. I *have* overcome one impossible situation after another. My life growing up was horrendous, *and* I've had extraordinary experiences that have completely transformed me, and made me the person I am today. Out of every negative situation have come many positive, healthy experiences and transformations because I've learned to be open, to look for, and to purposefully work for them. I am grateful that I've chosen to say yes to positive, healthy friendships with exceptional, honorable, loving, and kind people; I treasure and love them all. In a matter of a few seconds, these stories flash across my mind.

SURVIVAL

At age seven, half-brother began to sexually, physically, and emotionally torture and assault me many times a week. He'd come into my bedroom and rape me. No matter what I did, I could not stop him. I never knew when he'd explode into an insane rage. With one hand, he picked me up by the throat and shoved me as hard as he could against the wall; my feet dangled. He tightened his grip and kept threatening to put me through the wall; my feet kicked for dear life. His twisted smile and sadistic eyes found pleasure in torturing me; my life was being extinguished. Slowly, he released his grip, just enough to give me a wisp of air and a little bit of hope. Time after time, I thought his torment must be over, but he squeezed even harder. Slowly, he crushed my throat – I could no longer breathe. He was amused; playing with death was one of his sick ways of entertaining himself. My world went dark, and I experienced an extraordinary peace. Then, he'd let go, and I dropped like a rag doll. Frantically, I gasped for air as he walked out the room. This was one of his regular weapons in his arsenal of torture. Later, he violently yanked me, within an inch of his stone, cold face. His spit sprayed me as he threatened, "Don't tell anyone about this, or I'll kill you. If you do tell anybody, they'll take you away from our family, and you won't ever come back. Anyway, no one would believe you."

****

I not only survived the horrors of growing up; I learned to thrive – my healing was a process. I realized that I was not the weakling. Step by step, I developed a great inner strength that I didn't know was in me.

Immediately, I have a gut sense, my brain healing journey will be a step by step process; I absolutely need to trust my gut, to keep delving deeper into my inner awareness training, and to keep persevering forward, *no matter what*. I also need to remember the tools and other experiences of my powerful past, especially the positive, healthy, and loving people and situations. These experiences will open me to the next right step in my brain healing journey. (Here are three experiences. The next four chapters I will share more of the extraordinary positive transformations from my powerful past.)

At age seven, I did three things to stay alive. First, I spoke as little as possible, which is pretty funny because my nickname was Chatty Cathy. Hindsight is 20/20; now I know silence is where depravity exists. On the other hand, courage thrives by shining a light into the darkness and speaking the truth, even when afraid.

The second way I dealt with all the horrors was drinking beer, wine, and liqueurs. I saw adults drinking, having fun, and laughing. I thought drinking would make me feel better, and if I drank enough it would take me away from this hell. One night, my parents were having a party, after a while everyone moved into the kitchen. I stayed in the living room because someone had left a half glass of beer. I gulped the beer down, and immediately felt a warm glow inside. *I wanted more*. Floating into the kitchen, I grabbed another beer and guzzled it down, everyone laughed. Drinking was my escape. All my fears and worries instantly disappeared. I felt invincible and thought drinking made me tough enough to endure the horrors of my life in crazy land, my bio-family.

The third tool was my only positive, healthy tool; a love of nature. Nature was my safe haven and saving grace. When I explored the woods, I was at peace. I also believed that if I kept out of half-brother's way, maybe I could survive another day.

A wonderful memory of my youth comes to mind. On a cool, autumn day, I was walking in the woods when a pheasant sprung up by my feet and startled me. Each beat of his wings generated a rush of air that reverberated against my body. He was stunning and so close that it was easy to see his feathers: beautiful shades of brown, flecks of gold, and iridescent colors. Most notable was his instinct to survive. He gave me courage to survive; even though, I didn't know how. My next memory is one of my greatest gifts.

HOPE

Growing up, I thought everybody's life was like mine. That is until I experienced love, warmth, kindness, and safety. When I was seven to twelve years old, my little brother Richard and I visited my Aunt Sue and Uncle Phil's home for two weeks every summer. Richard and I were like sponges soaking up every morsel of love.

On a warm, sunny late afternoon, Aunt Sue called us kids to get ready for dinner. I was filled with excitement as I came downstairs – not dread – what a welcome and refreshing change. I followed the delicious aroma of beef bourguignon into the kitchen where my aunt gave me the special job of getting my uncle for dinner.

Enthusiastically, I flung the back door open. Before I hit the top step, I was greeted by the sights and smells of my uncle's magnificent garden; he's a master gardener. A plethora of exquisite rose bushes and an array of flowers, bushes, and trees surrounded their home. With each step, I was invigorated by a vibrant rainbow of hues: vivid reds to painted salmons, and sun-kissed yellows to blushing pinks. The exotic fragrances and abundant beauty caressed my senses and filled my soul. Once again, I had found my oasis in nature.

Enthralled by all the flowers and trees, I nearly forgot what I came outside to do. Looking to my left, I saw my uncle tending to his prize winning roses. He warmly welcomed me and introduced me to each rose bush he was caring for. Their home and sumptuous garden was a safe haven.

At the dinner table, my aunt and uncle's creations came

together. In the center was a vase of brilliant red roses accented with day lilies. I love the smell of flowers, especially day lilies. My aunt placed the steaming beef bourguignon with its rich, mouthwatering aroma to my left. The intermingling of the food, flowers, and this loving family nourished my hungry soul.

Before we ate, they always prayed, thanking God for the food and family. I didn't know how to pray, so I looked around and followed what everyone else did. Then, we sang the song, Amen, Amen which always lifted my heavy heart. I felt whole inside when we sang and even smiled. What a miracle – I smiled.

Finally, we ate and I savored all the sumptuous flavors. There was an ingredient in the food that I hadn't ever tasted before – love and kindness. Lively conversation filled the room, rather than the rage filled fights or worse, the deadly silence. Everyone talked about their day and what they had learned.

I was bathed in laughter, joy, and loving kindness. Something was happening inside me which was difficult to understand. I felt my Aunt Sue had become my real mom; even though, I knew she wasn't my biological mom. Inside, I felt a sense of peace and comfort. I had a mom who loved and cared for me.

Sunday morning everyone was getting ready for church. Sheepishly, I walked up to my aunt and said, "I don't have anything good to wear." My aunt's answer surprised me. "That's OK! God doesn't care what you're wearing." Her matter of fact words and reassuring tone comforted and profoundly affected me. A positive, healthy change was occurring within me. In that moment, I made a decision that forever transformed my life. One day, I too would live free, and be part of a loving, positive, healthy family.

****

The wonderful experiences at my aunt and uncle's home warms my heart and broadens my smile. Even in the midst of total despair and darkness, there is *always hope.* Love is always stronger than hate, sickness, or any other negative gunk – fear. It doesn't matter whether it's the horrors of my past, TBI, or anything else. *I need to keep persevering forward and to always have hope and love, no matter what.*

A NEGATIVE TRANSFORMS INTO A GREAT ASSET

*The focus of my book is my brain healing journey and the method I developed that completely healed and enhanced my brain better than before the TBI. For this reason, I will briefly touch upon my addiction to alcohol, my recovery process, and some of the tools I utilize which will also help me in my brain healing journey. If you want more information about recovery from addiction, please contact a qualified addiction counselor.

I treasured every moment at my aunt and uncle's home. They nourished my hungry soul and gave me hope. Unfortunately, I had to go back to crazy land, my bio family, and do everything I could to stay alive.

As I stated earlier, prior to my first visit to my aunt and uncle's home, alcohol was already a problem. At seven, I took my first drink, and immediately, alcohol turned on me; it became an obsession and began its inevitable destruction. I kept chasing that magical feeling of my first drink though I never, ever experienced it again. When I drank, I fit in, felt free, and whole, but it was only temporary. The agony of my life always returned. I continued to drink, searching for relief, only to find more misery, guilt, remorse, shame, and resentments. I was also always hyper-vigilant and barely slept; I never knew when I'd be attacked. Trying to drink away the pain was insane, but I didn't know any other way to deal with the rapes, torture, and horrors. As the saying goes, insanity is repeating the same thing, over and over again, and expecting different results.

At age twelve, I began having blackouts, but I didn't have a clue what was happening. One moment, I was drinking and it was late afternoon. The next moment, I woke up in bed; it was morning. I thought, I just forgot or had memory slips. In terror, I wondered what had happened. What did I do, and more importantly, what had been done to me? Although I was full of fear, I continued to drink because I could not stop.

School was my last safe haven. In sixth grade I made all "A's," this was the first time I had achieved such high marks. Proudly, I presented my report card to bio-mom, as I now call her, she barely looked at it, then berated me. From that moment I hated school and hated my life. **At age twelve I completely gave-up.**

On Sundays, Dad always cooked a delicious dinner. My job was to set the table, and my first priority was to grab the gallon jug of wine from the bottom cabinet closest to the back door. With pride I placed the wine in the middle of the table; then, set the rest of the table. One Sunday, my Aunt Dorothy was coming for dinner. I liked it when Aunt Dorothy came over because bio-mom was always on her best behavior. Inwardly, I chuckled at the *show* bio-mom always put on when she was out in public, when people came to visit, and when we visited other people. She smiled and was very pleasant – everything looked good on the outside. But, bio-mom had an absolute penchant for creating misery; it seemed to be her driving force. Bio-mom knew of the abuse, but she didn't stop it – she blamed me.

After I set the table, I watched Aunt Dorothy sit as far away as possible from the stove and counters. Later, she told me her secret. "When I sit here, I don't have to get up to get things because two people would have to move for me to get out." She leaned in a little closer. "All I have to do is to sit here, and enjoy all this delicious food." Her smile was as wide as a Cheshire cat, and her strategy was brilliant!

Before dinner was served, I was already drinking. Though I loved good food, I had trouble swallowing. At the time, I didn't understand it was because half-brother forced me to perform oral sex, among other horrendous things. While everyone else was eating, I was drinking one glass of wine after another. What little food I ate was forced down with wine.

I was draining another glass of wine, when Aunt Dorothy looked right at me and said, "You're drunk!" Everyone was startled; one of the unspoken truths was out in the open. While everyone else jumped up from the table and tried to escape, I lowered my glass and looked at Aunt Dorothy, which was unusual because I no longer looked directly at people. I thought about the people I'd seen drunk. Was I like them? That was my last memory, I blacked out. The next moment, it was Monday morning and bio-mom was yelling at me to get up for school. I hated Mondays, and now, I know why. I always had a hangover.

In ninth and tenth grade I was a "C" student. Half-brother moved out and the rapes stopped, but my life continued to be in physical danger. Even though I still didn't like school, didn't put in any more effort into studying, and I continued to drink, my grades skyrocketed to "A's" and "B's."

At eighteen, I was drinking every day, except on the Sundays when I couldn't get booze. I also suffered through the delirium tremors; DT's with the bugs crawling all over my skin, the snakes, and the little men with their pointy little hats leaping through the window and into the bedroom. I was also thrown out of just about every bar I drank at. Instead of taking responsibility for myself, I always blamed my drinking buddies for getting us thrown out. I never took responsibility for anything.

In my sick mind, I didn't think my drinking was that bad, compared to other people. However, over time, I had consistently lowered my standards of who had a worse problem with drinking than I. This way, I didn't have to take a look at my drinking. Though there were times I knew I was lying or BS myself.

My life was circling the toilet bowl, and I was the one who kept reaching up and flushing it away. I had become a Fuck Up from Fuck Up Land. My life sucked, and I hated myself. In my sick mind, I still thought booze was my best and only friend. There were times I remembered the wonderful experiences at my aunt and uncle's home. The sense of love, safety, and freedom drifted into consciousness. Instead of enjoying those magnificent memories, I drank even more to kill the memories because I knew I didn't deserve anything good.

The beginning of the end of my drinking occurred with a series of events at work. On a regular basis, a boss called me into his office and told me he wanted to throw me onto the floor and have his way with me. I knew he meant it. Somehow, each time, I got out of his office. At the time, I had no clue about sexual harassment and certainly didn't know how to deal with it.

I started having horrific flashbacks and nightmares of the rapes, tortures, and horrors of growing up. I told one of my drinking buddies, a 6' 7" guy, about that boss. He was furious and wanted to knock his lights out. Jokingly, we talked about killing him, then we switched tactics. We intently tried to figure a real solution to stop him, but we didn't come up with anything. Our conversation ended and I got drunk and blacked out as usual. Although no harm came to that boss, I was full of guilt, shame, and remorse for just thinking about hurting another human being. How could I even think about hurting someone after what I had been through? In my deluded state, I thought I would go to jail for what I thought.

I no longer considered myself a human being. I had lost my soul and knew there was no way I could get myself back. I felt as though I'd survived a war; I was completely hollow inside, only my skin held me together. The horrendous flashbacks and nightmares increased and continued to terrorize me.

The disease of addiction always gets worse without help. Alcoholism / addiction is a fixed fight, a slow form of suicide.

However, in every alcoholic's or addict's existence, there's at least one opportunity, usually more, to live sober and free. At twenty-two years old, I hit rock bottom – I was drinking to die. Somewhere inside, I knew I would not see my twenty-third birthday – if I continued to drink. Physically, I weighed a little over one hundred pounds, about fifty pounds less than my normal weight. I knew I needed to get and stay sober. But, in every cell of my being, I also knew that I could not stay sober, it was – impossible. I had tried everything I knew to stay sober, and each and every time, I utterly failed. In reality, I was a "want to, want to," a person who wants all the results, but won't do all the work to get those results. My entire life, I had quit most things I tried. If I did follow through with something, I didn't give it my best effort – except for drinking.

It was time to make a decision. Would I honestly face myself and stay sober? Or, would I continue spiraling down, into the dregs of non-existence? I thought of a sign I'd made recently. On graph paper, I had boldly printed.

Quitters Never Win!

Winners Never Quit!

I laughed at the word quit; the irony on so many levels didn't escape me. Instead of focusing on the negative aspect of quitting, something changed in me. I opened up and received what I will always call – the gift of desperation. I made a decision to stay sober, even though I had no idea how, and everything, absolutely everything, was against me. Unlike all the other times before, when I thought I wanted to stay sober, this time I had truly surrendered and was willing to do anything and everything to stay sober. My first day of sobriety was October 20, 1981, and I have been continuously sober since, one day at a time.

At the time, I thought hitting rock bottom and stopping drinking was the worst thing, ever. In hindsight, it was one of my best decisions. One of the first things I did was stop hanging out with my drinking buddies. I thought life would be boring and dull; I couldn't have been more wrong. I began to change direction by consciously looking for, and hanging out with new friends who were positive and caring, and to my surprise, I learned later that they were spiritual. My first close friend Tex (Janet) wasn't an alcoholic or an addict. I was shocked, Tex was a regular person, who happened to be a born-again Christian with a deep abiding faith. She didn't talk or preach about her faith, and she didn't try to change me. Her actions spoke louder than her words. To say I was hesitant to trust Tex and my other new friends would be a huge understatement. But, they didn't give up on me; they continued to love and be there for me. Tex provided the fertile soil for the seeds of unconditional love, kindness, and hope planted by Aunt Sue and Uncle Phil to grow.

The great conversations with Tex helped me to regain my voice and life. Slowly, very slowly, my world opened, as I learned how to do cool stuff sober: movies, dancing, softball, hanging out and supporting each other, goofing around, and having a great time. There were a few people, not my friends, who took bets that I could never, ever stay sober. Though their negativity bothered me, it was my new friends who helped me to keep focusing on the positives and what was working, I was staying sober.

Life was slowly improving. However, I still wanted and wished for a magic wand to keep me sober and to take away all the gunk of the past. But magic wands etc. are illusions existing only in the minds of people who won't do all the work to get all the results. In time, I would learn that living sober and free takes vigilance.

One thing that surprised me was I thought I didn't have a clue how to persevere. I quickly learned that *every person is an expert at persevering*. The only difference is the direction people are diligently pursuing. Alcoholics and addicts in the throes of addiction are experts at persevering backwards. We spend an enormous amount of energy, time, and money imprisoning ourselves in addiction. Whereas people, truly living in recovery, are focusing on: moving forward, cleaning up their past and their thinking, words, and lives, in order to live sober and free.

Very early in sobriety, I asked my friends for suggestions on how to stay sober and live free. Although they freely shared what helped them, I didn't listen to everything they said. Here are a few things that I heard. They talked about learning to be honest with themselves and others, cleaning up their past: their thinking, words, actions, and lives, and also having a relationship with a Higher Being. They said all of this wouldn't happen all at once, it was a step by step process. They said I could call this Higher Being, God, Allah, Buddha, nature, the great outdoors, or whatever worked for me. In the beginning of their sobriety, they didn't want to ask for help. But, they saw others, who had developed a relationship with a Higher Being, who were staying sober and enjoying life. They said in the beginning they prayed even though they didn't believe and certainly didn't have faith.

With time and effort, they were able to make the decision and take a leap into faith. They shared how their relationship with a Higher Being opened the door to an authentic relationship with themselves, then others. My friends had a sparkle in their eyes; their inner beauty shined from deep within. I watched them enjoy life, have fun, and help others – mostly by loving people. I also observed how they handled easy and difficult situations and dealt with their mistakes. When they got off track, they didn't run away or blame. They took responsibility for themselves, and to the best of their ability, corrected their missteps. Then, they redoubled their effort to be in harmony with themselves, with their faith, and with their ethics – they did all the work to get all the results.

My friends didn't talk about their faith unless I asked. They lived their faith; they epitomized the saying: Actions speak louder than words. They would not tell me what to believe. My friends understood, if you try to shove faith or anything else down a person's throat, they will throw up on your shoes, meaning: get resentful, mouthy, and balk. They said every person has to find their own way in life and in faith. If I wanted to know about their journey and what they do, they would share with me, but I had to ask. I didn't want to ask because I didn't want to appear weak. In reality, I was afraid. Yet, I desperately wanted someone to tell me what to do, and if it didn't work, I could blame them. To say that I was confused would be a huge understatement. My friends didn't tell me what to do; they weren't going down that unhealthy, negative road. The responsibility to ask for suggestions, help, and to do all the work to recover and live free – rested squarely on my shoulders.

One day, I was in so much pain that I asked my friends for suggestions. One suggestion was to put my sneakers way underneath my bed before I went to sleep. Since I was on my knees, it would be a good time to say thanks for another day of sobriety, one day at a time. In the morning, after I grabbed my sneakers, I could ask for help to stay sober, one day at a time. They said I could ask for help from the Power that helps them to stay sober, or anything else, as long as I didn't pray to myself or another human.

In absolute desperation, I began praying to stay sober. My first prayer was simple and filled with swear words. To whom or what I prayed to, I did not know and did not care. I got down on my knees to get back on my feet. Here's the cleaned up version. "Please, help me to stay sober today."

I learned two things from praying. First, day after day, it was a little easier to stay sober, which was a miracle beyond miracles! Second, kneeling on a hardwood floor hurts like hell. The success of my prayer experience was the beginning of a transformation. In time, I would add other prayers: to take away the obsession to drink, and turning over my will and life – thinking and all actions over to a Higher Being. I ended all my prayers with, "Thy will be done," in order to stomp on my ego with both feet. Although I was still many, many light years away from having faith, I couldn't deny that prayer was working.

It seemed like I was doing everything to stay sober and deal with the horrors of my past, but I knew I wasn't giving my best effort. Basically, I still thought I would never, ever be healed, and didn't deserve anything good, so why try. In time, I'd discover what was holding me back – fear. Despite being plagued by fear, I kept working on being healed. At the time, I didn't know I was about to face one of my biggest fears. Fortunately, my friend's love and my sobriety had given me a little bit of inner strength to face this fear.

My first spring sober, half-brother visited the family. I was living at the house, and I did everything to avoid him. Thinking I was safe, I went to the kitchen to get something to eat. I was shocked as I turned the corner. He was standing there stalking his prey – me. Time slowed and everything became crystal clear. I knew he was going to kill me. There was nowhere to run and nowhere to hide. In an instant, I made a new decision. I was going to live, *no matter what.* Inside, I experienced a surge of power that I had never felt before. Next to me on the stove was a heavy skillet. Before I could think, he lunged at me. I reached for the skillet and was about to pick it up when he hesitated. His upper body, arms, and hands swayed as he tried to attack me. Yet, his shoes seemed nailed to the floor. His upper body continued to sway back and forth. Fear was in his eyes, and his fear was intensifying. Without saying a word, he turned and flew out the back door. At the time, I had no idea that this was his last attempt on my life. However, for years I lived in fear that he would kill me. Initially, how I dealt with fear wasn't positive or healthy.

A little over one year sober, one day at a time, I moved into the YWCA ("Y") in Lowell, Massachusetts, a sober place for women in transition. I had my own room and thought living alone was one of the most brilliant decisions I had ever made. In my irrational thinking, I thought the cause of 90% of all problems was other people. Soon I would realize the real reason – my mind-set.

I was still tormented by flashbacks and nightmares. The horrors in my mind continued to intensify and became too much to bear. I made a decision and came up with a permanent solution to a temporary problem. I thought if I killed half-brother, then killed myself, I would be free of all the horrendous brutalities. This crazy idea led me to put myself into a mental health unit at the local hospital. In my sick mind, I called it the "Ha Ha Hilton" or "Cracker Factory."

My friends and mentors supported me and visited often. One day, Tex walked in and there was something different about her. There was a palpable, loving energy that came from inside and surrounding her. I had never experienced that before. Tex sat across from me and calmly said.

"Cathy, I don't want you to commit suicide. I want, and need you here."

She continued to look at me with pure love. In that moment, I understood that Tex and my other friends and mentors had always loved me. I was the one who had not let them in. The walls I built to protect me from harm had imprisoned me, and kept everyone who loved me from entering in. Tex's simple, caring, and profound loving words offered me a bridge to life and forever changed me. I made a decision to live, to redouble my efforts to attain emotional sobriety, and to transform my life.

Over the next few weeks, I took an honest look at how much time and effort I had put into living sober, cleaning up my past, and changing my thinking, words, and actions. Though I had worked hard, I absolutely knew I hadn't given my best effort. Although I hadn't picked up a drink for over a year, I was dry, not sober, and I was at a crossroads. Would I move forward, by honestly facing my fears in order to be healed and truly free? Or, was I going to be a "want to, want to," a person who talks on and on about how they need help, how they need to change, and say they'll do anything to change and be healed and free. But, they don't do all the work? In fact, they usually do very little work, if any.

It was time to make a decision and take action. Although I was scared to my core, I decided to do everything and anything to live sober, healthy, and free. Instantly, a passion rose within me. I wanted what my friends and mentors had: peace in my heart and mind, to enjoy each moment, and to be my true authentic self. I mustered up the courage and asked my mentors and friends for suggestions. They shared the same suggestions they'd offered before. This time, I listened intently, and shoved my pride where the sun don't shine; the part of my anatomy I sit upon. Here's a compilation of some of their suggestions.

"Cathy, stop playing the blame game – take responsibility for your self. No one can do the work for you. The responsibility to live sober and free always rests squarely on your shoulders. Rather than be overwhelmed with all your problems, take things – one at a time. Honestly deal with the task that's right in front of you, by focusing on what you can do, not on what you can't. You'll begin to realize that the vast majority of your problems are between your ears – your mind-set. By dealing with one problem at a time, you'll remove the self imposed protective prison that's handicapped and separated you, brick by brick. Your problems and wall won't come down in one fell swoop. You'll gain momentum by persevering, one task at a time.

This is a journey, not a destination. You will make mistakes, it's natural. Rather than kick your butt, use your energy to be honest, to learn from them, and to clean up your mistakes to the best of your ability. Fear will pop up, but don't feed the fear or anything negative. Face the fear as soon as it comes up. Be constructive by focusing on and feeding your self what is positive, healthy, and what's working. Also, be aware of what you're inputting into your life and mind. Listen, read, and watch things that you love and that inspire and encourage you. Finding out what floats your boat and what doesn't will be trial and error. Every person has to figure it out for themselves. Also, share what you've learned and experienced with others who ask, who truly want to be helped, and who do all the work to get all the results. Continue talking and hanging out with positive, healthy, and encouraging people who help others and fully enjoy life.

Doing all this on your own will be an enormous undertaking. However, every day you've made a decision to develop a relationship with a Higher Being, God, Buddha, Allah, Divine Source or whatever you want to call it. Keep growing in and with your relationship with your Source. Make it a priority. Do all the work to get all the results and your thinking, actions, and life will get and stay squared away. If you practice these suggestions, one day at a time, your life will be more rewarding, easier, and sweeter. You'll become a little more grateful, honest, caring, humble, and you'll want to help others. One day, you won't have to consciously think about doing these suggestions; they'll be a natural part of you."

I took their suggestions to heart, and began implementing them, except for one. I wasn't ready to seek a relationship with a Higher Source; though, I did continue to pray. I also thought, change would happen in one fell swoop, but that's backward thinking. When my thinking did get off-course and I made mistakes; I got back on track as soon as possible because I liked feeling good inside. It's funny, I always knew the right thing to do; people do. Little by little, it became natural to have a positive mind-set, be grateful, healthier, and happier. I really liked having my thinking and life squared away.

****

Reflecting on the beginning of my sobriety is encouraging me to keep persevering in my brain healing journey. **I will not give-up on myself like I did when I was twelve; I know where those decisions and actions will take me, and I'm not willing to go backwards. I need to have faith and trust myself.** I also need to stop listening to and feeding the negativity and impossibles coming from others and from my thinking. The next memory puts a huge smile on my face.

SAY YES TO LIFE

Around two years sober, an incident happened at the "Y" which forced me to find a temporary place to live. Fortunately, Tex's family; the Mackey's, Ginny (mom), Ned (dad), Tex, and her sister Lauren opened their loving home. They were very down to earth; in many ways, they reminded me of Aunt Sue and Uncle Phil. For two weeks, I was safe, cherished, respected, and loved. Another positive, healthy transformation had begun in me. Sometimes, well most times, healthy changes are not comfortable, including this one. However, positive transformations always blossom into wonderful experiences, as long as I'm open, look for, and purposefully work for the positive, healthy changes.

I returned to the "Y," and three days later, I began having a feeling which confounded me. I talked with one of my friends who helped me figure out that I was lonely. I absolutely did not like this new feeling. A long time ago, I decided the best thing was to live by myself and not to get close to people. Despite my old resolve, this new feeling of loneliness was more powerful. I asked a friend for suggestions, and was totally surprised by his answer. "Ask Ginny if you could live with them. Offer to pay what it costs at the Y." I was taken aback and asked, "What if she says no?" Quickly, he countered, "What if she says yes?" I thought of his response; then, I asked a question even though I didn't want an answer. "How would I ask her?" He smiled and said, "When you're ready, call and ask if she'll meet you for a cup of coffee. Say you'd like to talk with her."

Three days later, I came face to face with my thinking and a saying that summed it up. A coward dies a thousand deaths, but a brave person dies only once. In the past, I said no to opportunities, then blamed, complained, and gave all sorts of excuses. From not being lucky enough, to never, ever having opportunities or they weren't good enough, etc. In reality, I wanted everything to be easy and perfect. Basically, I didn't want to do the work. I also had a twisted sense of pride of being tough; I could do everything on my own.

I was at a crossroads; I was tired of existing as a coward and fear running my life. Instead of doing what I always did, I prayed for courage, and immediately started practicing what I was going to say to Ginny. The next day, as I walked to the pay phone upstairs in the "Y," I practiced and prayed. I called Ginny and said I wanted to talk with her, and asked if she would like to meet at Dunkin Donuts on Bridge Street in Lowell. She agreed, and we set up a day and time. I hung up the phone and let out a huge sigh of relief.

As the meeting with Ginny approached, fear erupted again. Rather than feed the fear, I kept praying, focusing on the positives, and what I was going to say. The day of the meeting, I was beyond nervous. Opening the door, I smelled the delicious aroma of coffee and donuts. I looked around. Ginny smiled at me, she was calmly sitting in a booth with a cup of coffee. I got a cup of coffee, sat across from her, and stared at the table. Thankfully, I had prayed beforehand. With my eyes glued to the table, I asked if I could live with them. Without missing a beat, Ginny said, "Yes!" The relief I felt as I looked up at Ginny was indescribable.

As I drove away, and over the next few days, I reflected on what had happened. *I walked up to this humongous wall of self-built fear. As I was about to face all the fears, the wall disappeared. By facing fear, I freed myself. Even if Ginny had said no, I would have still won and been freed because I faced the fear. Fear was only a self-made delusion – the problem was in my mind-set – what I focused on and fed. Fear and negativity had absolutely nothing to do with other people and situations. In that moment, I made two decisions – from that point forward, I would not let fear stop me, and that I would be a warrior of positive transformations. Although I made the decision to not let fear stop me,*

I needed to keep making the decision and consistently take positive actions. Again, my journey to freedom was a step by step process.

****

There are definitely common themes in my powerful past. I need to stop giving power to other people and *their* negative, hopeless beliefs about completely healing my brain, being reconnected, or anything else. I need to face the fear of not knowing how to liberate myself from the TBI, and trust that I will discover a solution. With my intention set, my next extraordinary life changing memory unfolds.

A DECISION TO RECEIVE UNCONDITIONAL LOVE

The Mackey's welcomed me into their loving home. But, I kept a safe distance and continued to always be hyper-vigilant. At the dinner table, I listened to healthy conversations and laughter as everyone shared about their day. I soaked everything in. Slowly, I gained weight though I was still severely underweight. In the morning, before work, Ginny and I would talk about having a hard time sleeping. She'd joke that we could do eight hours with one hand tied behind our backs; she was right. The Mackey's continued to love me, and without knowing it, a chink was appearing in my wall.

The center of activity was the kitchen. One night, after dinner, everyone cleared out of the kitchen like it was on fire, except for Ginny who continued washing the dishes. Bewildered, I looked around and didn't see anything wrong. I brought up my plate, cup, and utensils, and thanked Ginny for the meal. As I turned to walk away, Ginny calmly said.

"Cathy, I'd like to have a conversation with you. Please, have a seat."

Normally, my heart would race when someone said they wanted to talk with me: usually it meant something was wrong. For some reason, I was calm. At first, I chalked it up to the peaceful tone in Ginny's voice. As I sat down, I sensed a presence, a powerful Love that embraced me and exuded through the kitchen. Ginny continued washing the dishes and without looking at me said.

"Cathy, you think you know how to give. You know how to give money, and you know how to give presents. But, you really don't know how to give because you've never learned how to receive." She paused. "This is your time to receive."

While Ginny continued washing the dishes, this Love and her simple, profound words resonated deeper and deeper within me. My withered soul was being nourished. I made a decision to open and unlock my self-protective walls. Immediately, I received one of the greatest gifts of my life – unconditional love. Inside, I felt more whole, like I belonged. There's nothing to prove and nothing to do – I am loved. It didn't matter, that I'd been battered, abused, tortured, and had tried to self-destruct, or how hard I had worked to change my life through counseling, support groups, and books. The answer was not "out there" and it's not "in things." *The answers are always inside.*

Wrapped in a blanket of unconditional love, I began to thrive. Accepting love gave me hope which opened me to the possibilities of truly being healed. My dream of living with a positive, healthy, and loving family had come to fruition. Months passed, and I began having a desire to connect with a Higher Being, or whatever words worked for me. I didn't know how to explain it or why it was happening now and not earlier. Inside, it was the right time. I had faced my small-minded prejudices about the loving people of faith in my life. They had made a profound impression on me. They walked their talk, embodied love, were fully living their lives, and had a deep faith in their God, in themselves, in me, and in others. I talked with them about their faith. They let me know they were only a link, a bridge; they were not the source of this power. Once again, they said the responsibility of living sober, free, and being a person of faith – always rests squarely on my shoulders. Supported by love, I was ready to reach out and open the door. One weekend afternoon, I was in my room, on my knees praying to whom or what – I did not know. Ginny was walking by and gently asked, "What are you doing?" In a matter of fact manner, I told her, "I'm trying to find God." Ginny smiled and brightly said, "You will!" Her simple, upbeat answer and reassuring look encouraged me. Ginny walked down the hall, and I continued seeking God.

A few days later, I was home alone, sitting on the couch in the living room disheartened. I was still chained to my past and didn't know what to do. I began praying for help and direction. Almost immediately I became aware of a loving presence, like my experience in the kitchen with Ginny. It felt like a person had entered the room – exuding unconditional love. I looked to my right, towards the doorway. No one was there.

I looked forward and began praying again. A few seconds later, a shift occurred within me. The room seemed to open up. I was standing in sunlight – peace and love was in and enveloped me. The massive weight of my past began to lift. Somewhere deep inside, I knew everything would be ok – that I would be ok. *It was almost surreal to be unconditionally loved and flowing with Life. Until I realized, flowing with Life is how life is supposed to be lived. That night, for the first time since I was seven years old, I slept soundly.*

Having crossed the threshold into faith, I thought I'd be free of all the negative gunk of my past, especially my anger. I couldn't have been more wrong. My metamorphosis to faith was a good beginning, but I had more work ahead. It was time to step up and truly deal with my anger. I took a deep breath, exhaled, and decided to do whatever it took to be liberated from my past and from all my anger. I asked my friends and mentors. "How do I get over my anger?" All of them pretty much gave me the same answer.

"Cathy, every time a person gets angry – they're afraid." I rocked back on my heels. I prided myself on not being a fearful person. But, if this was true, I was like a neon light at night, announcing to the world that I was full of fear and that fear ruled my life. They continued.

"When you break down anger to its core, what's left is plain ole

fear. Most things people are afraid of aren't even real." Quickly, I remembered the time I faced the fear of asking Ginny to live with them and other situations since. By honestly walking up to and through fear, I experienced a profound life lesson – fear is an illusion. Being afraid wasn't the problem. Choosing to focus on and feed the fear, and letting it run my thinking and life was the problem. They continued to explain.

"Anger and fear are just emotions. What you decide to do with them will determine how you live your life. Cathy, think how far you've come, in a short amount of time. You're sober, and your thinking is getting more and more squared away. There's no way you could have done this by yourself. Are you trying to deal with fear by yourself? Or, are you asking your Divine Source etc. for help to get to the core of fear? Remember, you made a decision and every day you make a decision to give your will and life, your thinking and actions, to your Source. Either you trust and have faith, or you don't. It's like being pregnant; either you're pregnant or you're not. There is no such thing as being a little bit pregnant.

Also, fear will crop up, but just because you "feel" fear doesn't mean you're "in" fear. It means, you've gotten off-course, and you need to take positive actions to get your thinking on track. Ask for help to face and walk through the fear, and to keep moving forward: growing, changing, and thriving. In addition, being a person of faith doesn't mean you're weak, it means you have courage. Don't ever apologize for being a person of faith. Keep developing your relationship with Divine Source, be honest, and enjoy each moment. Also, share what you've learned: what works, what doesn't, and the solutions you've experienced because you faced fear with faith – love."

I perked up and said. "That's pretty simple, if people used these techniques, there'd be a lot less conflict in the world." My friends laughed. *"Cathy, **you're** the one asking, not other people. Applying this into **your** life will help **you** travel the road of life – happy, free, and with a peaceful mind. If other people want this, they'll have to do **all** the work to get **all** the results."*

I contemplated their suggestions, and immediately applied all of them. Little by little, my life began to positively transform.

Each time I faced fear with faith – love, I was becoming the person I had always wanted to be. With my thinking and life more squared away, it was time to face a big fear. Supported by love, I was able to be honest with myself and admit I was gay. Accepting I was gay helped me to sleep even better; I was finally being true with myself. However, I didn't want to tell the Mackey's, my strong born-again Christian family because I didn't want to get thrown out. Though, I knew if they rejected me, that was their problem, not mine.

Once again, I prayed for courage. I knew I needed to be honest to continue living sober and free. I walked into the kitchen and told Ginny and Tex that I was gay. They enthusiastically hugged and said they loved me! They told me they knew I was gay the moment they had met me, years before. This family – my family – cared, loved, and accepted me – their actions matched their words.

****

In a few seconds, my powerful past has once again helped me. I feel like a phoenix rising from the ashes. Out of every negative, I've experienced many positive transformations and blessings because I've learned to be open, to look for, and to purposefully work for positive, healthy change. I've not only survived my past, I've thrived beyond my wildest dreams.

My friendship with Tex and living with the Mackey's were two of the most pivotal experiences in my life which continues to influence me today. I wouldn't be on my brain healing journey if it wasn't for their love and support. As for living in faith – love and being a spiritual person, it's a way of life for me. There are many kinds of faith: faith in oneself, in an ideal, in another person, in an organization or group, and in a Higher Being or whatever words work for you. However, talking and writing about my spiritual path has been challenging. Personally, I prefer to let my actions speak louder than my words. I no more wear my faith on my sleeve, or talk about my faith than I talk about being gay: it's an integral part of who I am. However, if I didn't share a bit of this part of my journey, people wouldn't understand the powerful motivation for my brain healing journey. Pre-TBI I had an almost constant connection with Divine Source, but the thick, blurry glass wall prevents the vast majority of this connection. The powerful drive for liberating my self from the prison in my brain is to be *reconnected* with Divine Source, myself, the people I love, and the world. *I ache to be free and reconnected.*

6

FRIG IMPOSSIBLE

A fire of pure determination is being stoked in my gut. I need to find a solution, a path out of this quagmire of TBI. For over a year, I've felt like the ball in a pinball machine with every "No and Never" and "Impossible" knocking me around, but not out. So many times during this very long year I've thought, "Just tell me how to break through this prison in my brain? I'll do whatever it takes to free myself and be reconnected." But there isn't a roadmap on how to completely heal the brain, and waiting for someone else to develop a method, when they absolutely believe it's impossible. Well, that makes about as much sense as waiting for the – right time to get sober, to feel like being positive or do the right thing. It is absolutely nuts to wait for a magic pill, wand, or someone else to find a solution. If I keep traveling down that dead-end path, I will die imprisoned in my brain – that is not going to happen. *My spirit can only be broken if I make that decision, and my decision is to be free of this TBI.*

Why have I listened to experts who continuously say they know very little about the brain and that they're in the infancy of understanding the brain? Yet, they absolutely know it is

"Impossible" to heal the brain? I wouldn't expect a mechanic to repair an engine if they kept saying they didn't have the knowledge, the ability, or the tools to do the job. The best medical professionals don't have a solution to completely heal the TBI. Heck, they don't even have a clue. Just because everyone else believes with unequivocal certainty that it's impossible to heal the brain doesn't make it true. What it means is *they* think, believe, and accept that *they* can't do it and no one else can either.

I've reached the B. S. overload with people who focus on the negatives and the impossible. That's *their* defeatist mind-set, not mine. I will no longer believe or listen to others negativity. Frig *their* "no's and never's" and Frig *their* "impossible's." *Nothing is impossible. The only place impossible resides is in the mind, but not in mine! I am not going to let someone tell me what I can and cannot do. I will not be confined, defined, or controlled by anyone or anything, including TBI.*

The responsibility to be free of this prison in my brain rests squarely on my shoulders. From this moment forward, TBI is just like any other obstacle I've faced. I will overcome this TBI not by going through the walls others continue to build. I will find a way to rise up and break through the thick, blurry glass prison in my brain.

People have no clue what I'm made of; there are no tests to measure my determination and how hard I'll work to rise above whatever obstacles are in the way. Whatever people say I'm not able to do, I will do all that and more. My job is not to prove other people wrong and me right, that would be foolish and a waste of my precious time and energy. Instead, I'll use other people's doubts, negativity, and pessimistic outlook as added motivation. Rather than just listening when people are speaking *their* "no's and never's" and "impossible's," I will smile, nod my head up and down, and inwardly cheer. 'I'm from Missouri. Fucking watch me!' I laugh at my choice of states; although I'm from Massachusetts, Missouri rhymes better.

Having a TBI doesn't mean I have to have a weak ass mind-set and I'm not able to have fun. I will have a strong, positive, healthy attitude. I will enjoy each step in my brain healing journey, and I will keep persevering forward, *no matter what*. Again, it doesn't matter that there isn't a guide or book, not even a pamphlet to show me how to liberate myself from the thick, blurry glass wall. TBI is no longer a problem; it is an opportunity. I am a thriver and I will succeed.

Intentionally, I set my course. I will discover a solution to TBI; I will completely recover, be reconnected, and be better than before – no matter what! I must continue focusing on what has always worked; delving deeper into my inner awareness training. Immediately, in my mind's eye, my forever fall in the never-ending hole stops. I stand up, dust myself off, and begin climbing in utter darkness. Deep in my gut, I absolutely know I will discover new techniques and a method that will completely heal and enhance my brain better than before the TBI – my actions will speak louder than my words!

MAKING MY
BRAIN SMART

Before heading to the rehabilitation hospital, I make one more decision – I will not tell anyone about my resolution to completely heal and enhance my brain better than before the TBI. I know if I tell the rehab staff or anyone else that I'm going to develop a solution to completely heal my brain; in a heartbeat they'll send me to counseling because I haven't "accepted" my disability. Even a little well-intentioned concern could take me off course, and that's something I'm not willing to risk. With this decision, I have entered what I call; my quiet determination mode.

Enthusiastically, I tell my rehab team that I am going to college and will do well! They look at each another. Inwardly, I sense three things: they're skeptical, they admire my spunk, and they're not going to steer me in another direction. They advise me to attend Northeastern University because of their great department that provides note takers and other help for people with disabilities. Next, they change the direction of some therapies. I will learn study skills and more organizational skills etc. to prepare me for college.

The first mountain I face is, of course, in speech therapy where my writing skills will be evaluated. The speech therapist asks me to write a sentence, and walks away to deal with some papers on her desk. I stare at the blank sheet of paper. I have no idea how to write a sentence. I can point in a book to a sentence. I know it starts with a capital letter and ends with a period; I remember being taught this in elementary school. I have memories and some knowledge, but I don't have the skill to write a sentence. My heart is beating faster and my entire body is sweating; it feels like the walls in the room are closing in. Sheepishly I admit that I don't know how to write a sentence. Without looking, the speech therapist says a little perturbed. "Sure you do; now come on, write a sentence." With all the will I can muster, I focus as hard as I can, but I still don't know how to write a sentence. Finally, the speech therapist sits down, leans in, and looks deep into my eyes. Confusing energy is exuding from her. Next, I notice her stunned look; I don't think she knows what to do with me. She keeps asking me to write a sentence while I remember the "one-year rule" all the professionals have tried to pound into me. After one year, don't expect any improvement with your brain. It's been about a year since the accident. Is this my defeat? NO. Quitters Never Win. Winners Never Quit! *The only place impossible resides is in the mind, but not in mine. I will not give up on myself. I will keep striving and I will succeed – no matter what!*

7

A NEW
APPROACH AND A
MAMMOTH STEP
IN MY BRAIN
HEALING
JOURNEY

I'm sent to a specialized speech therapist at rehab who is very calm, even-keeled, down to earth, and patient. I continue working diligently using all the rehab techniques, but I still don't know how to write a sentence.

Rather than get frustrated, I take a deep breath and slowly exhale. Almost immediately, I get a very strong gut sense. *I need to focus inside – specifically, to my right inner arm and how my muscles, joints, and other parts move. Even though this doesn't make sense, I make a decision to follow my gut; again, I'd be a fool not to.*

Reaching for the pen, I immediately become aware of a muscle lengthening in my right upper arm. Next, I'm aware of a muscle in my lower arm, while continuing to be aware of the upper muscle. Then, I notice my elbow joint is moving like a hinge. SIMULTANEOUSLY, I'm aware of all three inner movements; the two muscles and elbow, and for the First Time since the TBI, I'm Reconnecting to parts of my Inner Body and I'm a tiny bit clearer! I have a gut sense that this is my first step in intentionally making Reconnections to my inner body! I love my inner awareness and brain healing training!

I grasp the blue rubber triangle cushion on the pen. Immediately, I'm Simultaneously aware of smaller muscles and joints etc. in my right hand and fingers, and the previous two muscles and elbow in my arm. Wow, another step in how to delve deeper into my inner awareness training: being aware of previous and new muscles, joints, etc. Inside, I search for the correct hand position – a layer of fog lifts and I'm a tiny bit clearer. I also feel like I'm getting lost inside my body. Until I realize – being aware of muscles and joints, etc. is the same as being aware of how my inner body responds to people and situations in the foreign outside world. I calm down and continue being aware of my muscles, joints, etc. Next, I do an experiment. I stop being aware of my inner body, and I completely flounder. I've lost my new-found clarity and reconnections.

I have a huge gut sense to focus most of my attention on a muscle in my right upper arm and how it is moving. Immediately, I switch my inner awareness; to be clear, I'm not physically getting closer to my arm. The best way I can explain this is it feels like looking through a long-range lens in a camera as it zooms in to a specific muscle. By focusing on one muscle, my inner awareness naturally deepens and I experience – another level of clarity. I'm also starting to understand what a sentence is and how to write it. What's interesting is that while I'm so purposefully aware of this one muscle, I'm unable to stay aware of the other muscles and joints, etc. moving in my arm, hand, and fingers; it's like they're out of focus. Intentionally, I widen my awareness to my entire inner arm, hand, and fingers. Immediately, I'm aware of the muscles, joints, etc. moving. I have entered a whole other world and it's – inside me!

Before I put pen to paper, I take a moment to make sure I stay aware of the muscles and joints, etc. in my right arm, hand, and fingers while writing. The pen moves toward the paper; I'm aware of new smaller muscles, joints, and the previous parts of my inner body, but I don't know their names. Should I learn the foreign outside world names of all these inner body parts? No, I have a strong gut sense that it will be a colossal waste of time and effort and a superficial, dead-end path which would only feed my ego.

*The pen touches the paper and I write a few words. Although I'm writing, the vast majority of my awareness is in the movements inside my inner arm, hand, and fingers. Simultaneously, I'm aware of new and previously discovered muscles, joints, etc., and I'm beginning to experience their inner connections, but I don't understand how the inner connections are moving. I smile. It doesn't matter because the concept of a sentence and how to write it is beginning to connect and it's happening from the – inside out. I'm flabbergasted. I don't have to understand the inner connections; I just need to be aware of how my inner body is moving, connecting, and responding – for the outside task of writing a sentence to improve! Trying to write a sentence by being aware of my inner body feels weird, good, and even a little bit natural. I'm not sure how to explain this and it may not make sense to some people. **I believe to truly understand my inner awareness and brain healing training, it needs to be personally experienced; otherwise, it is just another outside technique which will not work.***

I focus deeper into all the movements of my inner arm, hand, and fingers, and again, my inner awareness naturally deepens. The muscles and joints, etc. seem to be moving as one; though, it's challenging to pay attention to all the inner movements. I decide to focus to a single muscle. When I'm aware of one muscle, I expand my focus to a couple of muscles. Again, my inner awareness naturally deepens to a whole new level, and I'm able to write a sentence and understand from the – inside out, what I've done! In only a few minutes, I've become aware of a single muscle, then other muscles, joints, etc. which, step by step, helped me to delve deeper into my inner awareness training, and now, I'm able to write a sentence. What else can I do! I celebrate this off the charts, phenomenal achievement mostly on the inside and I'm not sure why.

Step by step, it's getting easier and easier to delve deeper into my inner awareness by zooming in then widening my inner awareness to all the muscles, joints etc. and how they are moving while writing. My inner awareness training is now play and beyond fun! I continue being aware of my inner body and it's pretty easy to write a paragraph. Inwardly, I celebrate conquering another gargantuan mountain; I wrote a sentence then a paragraph – what else can I do!

I decide to do another experiment. I focus only on the outer technique of writing – without being aware of my inner body. Once more, I completely flounder; all the progress I've made with writing, clarity, and focus is lost. This is a no-brainer; I must continue delving deeper into my precious inner awareness training to succeed.

I decide to take stock of my brain healing journey. For the first time since the TBI, I'm experiencing significant progress in three areas, but they're not happening at the same rate. First, my inner awareness has greatly increased my ability to focus to my inner body. Second, my outer focus on tasks has improved about half as much as my inner awareness, yet I'm able to write a sentence and paragraph, and I'm clearer. Third, my energy level has only slightly improved. I'm not sure why my progress is occurring at a three-tiered rate, but I really don't care because I am finally making real progress and my brain healing journey has momentum. I love my inner awareness training. I celebrate all my triumphs mostly on the inside, and again, I'm not sure why. What I do know is that the outside techniques of picking up a pen, finding the correct hand position, and writing are not the solution; they are only a means of delving deeper into my precious inner awareness training.

Its spring 1990, and I've signed up for one class at Northeastern University while continuing all my therapies at rehab. This afternoon I head out to my first class; I am excited and a little nervous. *I put on my backpack and immediately, I'm aware of new and previously discovered muscles and joints, etc. in my shoulders, arms, back, and legs. I'm also a tiny bit clearer – again, from the inside out. Each time, I become aware of a new part of my inner body while being aware of the previous areas; my inner awareness improves and a layer of fog lifts. In addition, I'm sleeping a little, little less, and my ability to do tasks in the foreign outside world continues to slightly improve.*

I arrive at the university exhausted, and find a quiet area to rest; it takes a lot of energy traveling to school. My watch alarm goes off, and I think about how much I need to sleep. My powerful motivation to completely heal and enhance my brain better than before gets me up. I take a deep breath, exhale, and try to wake up from the nap and the TBI. I sort of wake up from the nap, but nothing I do can break through the prison in my brain.

Class begins and I'm grateful that the university has provided a note-taker and that I can use my audio tape recorder to record the class. In addition, when I take a test, I'm able to go into a quiet room by myself and take as much time as needed. The professor is talking, and I'm diligently trying to follow her, but I'm not able to keep up. I'm about six steps behind. *Rather than get frustrated, I focus on what I can do. I become aware of my inner body, and I'm shocked – it's a little bit easier to pay attention and understand the professor. Maybe if I write notes during class, it will help me delve deeper into my inner awareness training. Who knows? Two sets of notes might get the information deeper into my brain. While reaching for and grasping the blue rubber triangle cushion on my pen, I become aware of muscles, joints, etc., which improves my inner focus, and in turn sharpens my outer focus, ever so slightly. My energy level also increases, but it's only minutely. I'm still not sure why my improvements are happening at a three-tiered rate. Although writing isn't as easy with the professor talking, I sense adding a task is a good way to improve my inner awareness, and it does.*

Class ends and the note-taker hands me her notes. Quickly, I look at her neat, in depth notes. In my broken speech, I thank her for taking the time to help me. Exuding from her is calm, compassionate energy and pride. The note-taker smiles, I believe she understands my sentiment.

Slinging my backpack over my shoulder, I'm aware of my very tired muscles, and the exhaustion is overwhelming. I leave the building, and at the top of the stairs, I begin searching for Dad in the parking lot. Finally, I see him waving; he's right in front me. I open the passenger door of my truck, which I'm still not able to drive and slump into the seat.

For the next three days, I recover from class while going to therapies at rehab. The next four days, I spend countless hours reading, listening to my audio tapes, writing and re-writing notes to get the information into my brain, and of course going to rehab. I wish I didn't have to sleep so much, but wishing won't get the job done. I need to make my brain smart so I can liberate myself, completely heal my brain, and be reconnected.

While studying, I do other experiments. Instead of using my right dominant hand with the wrist brace; again, my wrist was broken during the accident, I use my non-dominant left healthy hand to write a sentence. Immediately, I'm aware of new muscles and joints, etc. in my left arm, hand and fingers, while also being aware of previously discovered areas of my inner body, and I'm a tiny bit clearer and focused. Although my handwriting looks like chicken scratch, step by step, my inner awareness naturally deepens. Using my left hand, I press different buttons on my audio tape recorder; immediately, I'm aware of my inner left shoulder, more precisely my upper, inner left shoulder, and again, I'm a little clearer and focused! **This is huge – with each new inner awareness I make a new connection or reconnection in my body, and my ability to focus to my inner body improves; then, and only then, does my outer focus on tasks in the foreign outside world improve. Finally, my brain healing journey has momentum.**

I continue working diligently at school and rehab, and I receive an "A" for my first class – Yeaha! In the fall semester, I take two classes and receive an "A" and a "B+." *There is no doubt, without my inner awareness training, I would be back in drool land.* I continue taking classes, many are in Boston, and I have to take buses, trains, and trolleys to get to school. In order to deal with the deafening, screeching noises from all the different transportation as it stops and makes turns; I use headphones to listen to uplifting music like "Life Is Good" by Livingston Taylor.

The ever-changing movement from all the transportation helps me delve deeper into my precious inner awareness training. While being jostled, I become aware of new parts of my inner body. What's most interesting is because the movements are different than putting on a backpack, writing, etc. I'm experiencing new and deeper levels of inner awareness with my new and previously discovered muscles, joints, etc. Step by step, my inner awareness, then outer focus, and energy level increases, and my ability to do tasks in the foreign outside world improve.

However, I'm expending a lot of energy traveling to school in Boston and attending class. It's challenging to accept that I need help to get back to the house. Dad understands my tremendous desire to succeed and is also concerned for my safety at night. He works a full day in Cambridge, drives about forty minutes to the house, eats dinner, and watches the first part of whatever game is on. Then, he drives another forty minutes, all the way into Boston to pick me up at Northeastern. As I get in my truck, which I still can't drive, I try to remember to thank him for driving and always helping me. I figure if I thank him right away, I'll have a better chance of remembering. If I thank him later, that's cool an extra thanks is always good. The drive back becomes our time to connect and listen to the game. I am very thankful for Dad's compassion, patience, support, and positive attitude; he doesn't ever expect anything in return. Dad inspires me to be of service to others.

I continue delving deeper into my precious inner awareness training and it pays off enormously. In the 1990 – 1991 school year, I make the Dean's List! I am in shock, and Dad is prouder than a peacock. My phenomenal, off the charts improvements from my *inner awareness and brain healing training* are not just in school.

The first of the month is about to roll around, and that evening Dad writes a check to rehab and reminds me to give the check to the nice business woman. Early afternoon, the next day, I enter rehab with a sense of pride. Before crossing the threshold of the business office, I take a deep breath which calms me. I make eye contact with the nice business woman and proudly present her the check! What a miracle! On my own, I remembered to give her the check. I also now understand that money and the check ensures that I can continue going to rehab. Inwardly, I celebrate!

Finally, I get the okay from rehab to use the stove and apply for my driver license, Yeaha! The freedom behind the wheel as I practice in empty parking lots with Dad is exhilarating. I love my inner awareness training and brain healing journey!

The day arrives for my driving test, and Dad somehow figures a way to sit in the backseat. He talks with the officer about last night's game and other sports. I know what he's doing; he's trying to distract the officer. He's also giving me hints through the rear view mirror. We smile at each other; then, he motions for me to pay attention to the road. With ease I pass my driving test, and I am absolutely thrilled; once again, my inner awareness training pays off handsomely. I take the privilege of my license seriously; I only drive on really good days. Unfortunately, those days don't happen as often as I would like. On the days I do drive, I thoroughly enjoy each and every moment – Yeaha!

More time passes; it's been about two years since I started at rehab, and my next doctor's appointment I'm told there's nothing more rehab can do. Initially I'm little surprised, but quickly change my focus. *I will keep delving deeper into the only thing that's working – my precious inner awareness training. I also continue going to school and do very well. I chalk up all my outstanding progress and accomplishments to my #1 brain healing technique – my inner awareness training; it is an extraordinary technique that keeps on giving!*

THIS TRAIL ENDS
TRIUMPHS AND
PLATEAUS
LATE SPRING
1992

It's been about three and half years since the TBI, and my academic achievements are off the charts awesome.

Spring Quarter 1990

- History American Indians   A

Fall Quarter 1990

- American Sign Language   B+

- Earth Science   A

Spring Quarter 1991

- Intermediate Sign Language   B+

- Elementary Grammar   *

- Intro Psychology   A

Fall Quarter 1991

- Elementary Writing   * (changed to B+)

Winter Quarter 1991

- American Sign Language   B

- Data Processing   A

- Intro Psychology   A

Spring Quarter 1992

- Socl Psychology   A

But, and it is a big but, there is a downside to my outside success. I can immediately regurgitate information, but I cannot retain it. I'm also light years away from where I was pre-TBI. While other people focus on my remarkable outside success in their foreign outside world, they are totally missing the point. *I've plateau in my inner awareness training and brain healing journey. Also, there isn't a dent, not even a nick in the thick, blurry glass wall. If I continue going to school, I'll eventually have a degree – a piece of paper which will not liberate me from the prison in my brain.* Although rehab and the university are dead-end paths for completely healing my brain, I don't think of them as failures. I've learned so many tools; *more importantly, I know what doesn't work.* Like Humpty Dumpty where all the kings horses and all the kings men:' rehab, doctors, therapists, and higher education – *nothing outside the thick, blurry glass prison wall has been able to put me back together again.*

On the upside, it's been easy, fun, and so natural to, step by step, delve deeper into my inner awareness and brain healing training; they are the sole reason for ALL my extraordinary triumphs, and they ALL have occurred from the – inside out. However, without a map or even a clue as to what direction to take to continue delving deeper into my precious inner awareness training, I can feel myself getting discouraged. I decide to change my mind-set and think about my future. After I've liberated myself and have been reconnected, I hope to teach people, *in person*, everything I've experienced, discovered, and developed in my brain healing journey, especially my precious inner awareness training, because reading or talking about my method would be absolutely incomplete. With the fire in my belly re-stoked, I resolutely decide to keep delving deeper into my inner awareness and developing my brain healing training. I will discover a solution to the TBI. My search continues!

PART 2

8

MOVING TOWARD A NEW PATH EARLY SUMMER 1992

I need to discover another way to delve deeper into my precious inner awareness training. If I don't I'll stagnate, start heading backwards, and will die imprisoned in my brain. Although I don't know what that pathway is, in my gut I know my next right step is to leave Massachusetts. Though I'm torn, the thought of leaving everything I've ever known: friends and family, especially Dad is almost too much to bear. I know moving is the right decision, but trying to set up housekeeping is the fear of the unknown. Instead of feeding the fear, I decide to trust my gut; again, I'd be a fool not to.

I've always wanted to live out West; I love wide open spaces and being around horses makes my heart sing. As a matter of fact, I haven't ever liked the fast paced, citified side of Massachusetts.

My partner, who is more of a friend than a partner, will be moving with me, and she needs to find a college to continue her studies. As for me, I know higher education is a dead-end path for completely healing my brain, but I have a gut sense to check-out schools. Hopefully following through with this leg work will lead to the next step in delving deeper into my inner awareness training. After much research, we visit Colorado; the people are friendly, the pace is great, and I have many wonderful experiences. Colorado not only fits all of our needs, in my gut I know it's the next right step in my journey.

There are many parties with people wishing us well and many sad goodbyes, but I'm dreading the toughest goodbye of all, my Dad. The day comes to leave and before Dad and I hug, we both start crying like babies; I've never seen him cry. I keep trying to leave, but we keep crying, hugging, and saying how much we love each other. After many failed attempts, I finally leave. The sound of the door closing feels like a part of me is being ripped apart. After a few miles, I turn around. Dad opens the door and we start crying all over again. I leave again, and this time, there's no turning back. For two days an ocean of tears pour out of me; then, I stop crying; it feels like I ran out of tears.

Slowly, I get settled into my new life. I'm living two streets from an open space hiking area in the stunning foothills of Boulder, Colorado. I look out the west window and gaze at Dakota Ridge; out the south window, I admire the profile of the Flatirons. Every time I look at the gorgeous foothills and magnificent Rocky Mountains, I am astounded by all the beauty.

I adopt a dog from the Humane Society; she's a nine month old black lab, border collie mix or so the vet thinks. I take her for regular walks, and when I'm up for it, we do short hikes. The first month I call her about twenty-five different names ranging from Amazing Raison to Thumper because of how loud her tail wags when she's lying on the floor. One day, I call her Maja and the name fits, but I'm not sure how to spell her name. I announce a spelling contest and a few days later the winner is declared; one of my friends had a grandmother whose name was Maja.

Summer turns into autumn and the Aspen trees turn gold. For some reason I've been feeling even more tired; this increase in fatigue started when I was living in Massachusetts. Instead of taking multiple classes at the University of Colorado, I'm only taking one. But, my heart is not into school; it's a dead-end path for completely healing my brain. I am also very disappointed with the department that helps people with disabilities. Rather than focus on the negatives, I decide to change my mind-set. The office for people with disabilities at Northeastern University was awesome.

Dad visits for Thanksgiving and falls in love with Colorado. Before he heads home, a plan is made to go to Massachusetts for the holidays, and it's a great visit. Winter takes hold and I'm feeling extremely exhausted. In February of 1993, after many doctors appointments, I'm diagnosed with cancer; Non-Hodgkin's lymphoma. My emotions are running the gamut. In an instant, I've gone from living one of my dreams – living out West – to wondering if I'm going to die. I've been through so much: a TBI, being raped and tortured growing up, and now I have cancer. WHY ME! This isn't fair! Why do I have to get friggin cancer! I deserve a break! Then, I get really afraid that I'm not going to do all the things I was placed on this earth to do, even though I don't know what they are. A few days later, I decide to stop feeding the fears and reset my attitude which ends my pity party. Next, I decide to put on hold my search for developing a solution to the TBI, and I stop going to school. My focus must be on getting this gunk out of my body, and finding ways to deal with the new obstacles of nausea, even more exhaustion, and pain from the radiation treatments.

Once the initial shock of being diagnosed with cancer wears off, I begin to wonder about the *coincidence* of cancer on my neck and in my mouth, and all the times I was strangled and almost died, and the forced oral sex. Although I don't think it's a fluke, now is not the time to look backwards. I need to put all my resources on getting healthy.

The radiation treatments are adding up and eating is a chore.

One day, I'm craving a certain food, and the next day, I'm repulsed by the sight or smell of it. A week later, everything tastes like metal. In addition, my salivary glands are getting burnt to a crisp, which means in time, my teeth will be severely effected. To help deal with all the emotions and everything else, we start attending a cancer support group in Boulder. I meet great people in the group; we laugh, cry, and use gallows humor to deal with all the challenges and unknowns. But, every night after the meeting, I toss and turn in bed; whirling in my mind are thoughts of sickness and death. In the morning, I feel like I've wrestled a powerful faceless opponent who always gets the upper hand.

Consciously, I lift my spirit by gazing at the gorgeous foothills and the beautiful flowers, trees, and bushes beginning to bloom in the front yard. The splendor in front of me takes my mind off how yucky I feel. I'm also watching a lot of T.V. One day, I'm lying down, flipping channels, and feeling like the cat dragged me in and puked on me. Suddenly, I stop channel surfing, sit straight up, and watch a commercial for the old Kung Fu TV show. My spirit is awakened; the show was a positive influence and helped me deal with all the horrors growing up. They announce the entire series will be airing Monday through Friday in the afternoon. After watching a few shows, I'm inspired. Maybe one day I'll feel better. Then, I can continue my brain healing journey, discover a solution to the TBI, and once again I'll be healthy, intelligent, athletic, free, and reconnected.

MAKING A
DECISION TO LIVE
LIFE FULLY
SUMMER 1993

The radiation treatments have ended and death is all around me; I am in 'No Man's Land.' In six weeks, six people have died from cancer – four are friends and two are family. Out of all of the devastating losses, Ginny Mackey's death rocks me to the core. Am I next? While wondering if the cancer is in remission, I experience a new kind of agony – waiting for test results. 'No Man's Land' is no way to live.

Weeks later I receive a clean bill of health. I'm ecstatic and grateful to be alive, and I also feel guilty. I know I'm experiencing survivor's guilt, but this knowledge doesn't change how I feel. I go into a very quiet and deep introspective period; it feels like I've entered a cave to lick my wounds. I know I'm depressed, but this is vastly different than anything I've experienced. For the first time in my life, I'm pondering what life is all about? Why am I here? What are my life purposes? What does it really mean to be alive, living life fully, and enjoying each moment?

At times, the massive grief tries to swallow me up, and I have to intentionally focus on breathing in and out, and putting one foot in front of another, especially when I don't want to. Though I push myself to be physically active, the massive exhaustion, pain, and grief is limiting me. Thankfully, my love of nature and

Maja the wonder pup, one of her nicknames, slowly gets me moving. I've started calling all animals "pup," no matter there age: squirrels, birds, cats, dogs, raccoons, and coyotes. It puts a smile on my face to call them pup, and these days I'm doing everything I can to lift my spirit.

One of my mentors calls, and as always, the conversation is wonderful. After a few minutes, my thinking starts circling the toilet bowl with the "what ifs," "how comes," and "why me's?' My friend gently explains that changing her focus helped her through the dark times. I'm thankful my mentors know me well and don't give advice without being asked. I shift my focus and ask if she has any suggestions. Calmly she shares, "Next time you go out to the store buy a roll of lifesavers and carry them in your pocket. It may sound strange, but each time you reach into your pocket and touch the lifesavers you'll be reminded that all things pass with time. Grief, like life is not static. One day, the grief will subside, as it always has, and you'll be surprised by the sound of laughter coming from you." My first thought is she is absolutely nuts. My second thought is that I need to be open because I don't want to continue feeling awful, negative – full of fear. I ask her how to deal with all the loss and guilt. Her question shocks me. "Would your loved ones want you to be miserable, unhappy, guilty, depressed, and lost?" "No." As the word "no" comes out of my mouth, a shift occurs within me. Inside, I'm experiencing a slight glimmer of hope. Rather than seeing all the devastating losses and facing my own death as a whole bunch of negative stumbling blocks, I see everything as stepping stones. Maybe one day, I'll again be seeking; then, develop a solution to the TBI, which will free and reconnect me with Divine Source, myself, the people I love, and the world; this is what my loved ones would want.

I follow through with my friend's unusual suggestion; I buy a roll of lifesavers and put them in my front jean pocket. Each time I touch the candy I'm comforted. This simple package of candy helps me symbolize the preciousness of life, and in time, I will be completely healed. For years to come, I'll share this precious story and give many rolls of lifesavers to people going through challenging times. Many will share how the story and lifesavers comforted and helped them too.

A few mornings later, I'm upstairs looking at the apple tree in the side yard. The sparrows are having their usual squabble while other birds and wildlife search for breakfast. I think to myself; you get what you focus on. I become aware that my body is being warmed by the sun streaming through the east window. I look up and catch sight of the stunning foothills. Once again, focusing on the beauty of nature is creating a little light in the darkness. The next moment, I drift to the past. A few seconds later, I project into the future. The intensity of all the massive losses, grief, and pain draws me into the darkness – it hurts to breathe. Slowly, I consciously inhale. As I'm exhaling, I have a gut sense. Life is to be enjoyed and celebrated – fully treasure the gifts of each moment and the people in my life.

Purposefully, I change my mind-set by focusing on the dreams I had as a kid. Growing up, I loved working with wood, being in nature, and the thought of doing Kung Fu one day. Without hesitating I make a life-altering decision. I will do all the things I love, and I will live my life fully – *no matter what*. What about the TBI? The thick, blurry glass prison in my brain is still blocking me from everything I want and need to do. In every sense of the word, I am at a crossroads.

ACUPUNCTURE - A WHOLE NEW WORLD

A friend from the cancer support group suggests I try acupuncture and recommends an acupuncturist whom she trusts. Although it's supposed to take several months to get an appointment, my friend speeds up the process. I've never done acupuncture before and don't know what to expect. I open the door to the acupuncture office and cross the threshold into another world. The room is decorated with exquisite Chinese paintings, scrolls, and thriving plants. On one wall are big beautiful wooden drawers filled with herbs and other medicine from China. The waiting room is quiet, like other doctors' offices; however, there's a sense of peace in here that helps ease some of my apprehension.

It is 1993, acupuncture is still illegal in many states, and the vast majority of medical professionals believe it is voodoo. Instead of focusing on others' negativity, I decide to have an open mind and examine the facts. Acupuncture has been around for thousands of years while Western medicine has been around a few hundred years. What have I got to lose by checking out acupuncture, and who knows where this path will lead?

A petite Chinese woman appears and politely introduces herself. "My name is Yao please come in." Yao takes a thorough medical history and *takes my pulse on both wrists*. Checking my pulse is very different from Western medicine. In time, I'll learn that the *pulse method* checks my organs, energy level, whether my body is balanced, and so much more. She also looks at my tongue; I do not know why – I have much to learn about acupuncture.

Yao asks me to lie down and adjusts the pillow until my head is perfectly, gently supported. On the wall to my left are drawings of the human body with numbers and Chinese lettering; each character has a dot next to it. Yao explains that these are acupuncture points, and she'll be inserting needles in different places to help balance and heal me. Yao shows me an acupuncture needle which is fascinating. The lower third of the needle is a very thin wire which is quite flexible. The middle is slightly thicker, and at the top the wire coils into an interesting woven knot. Though I'm not fond of needles, I am very eager to experience how acupuncture works.

Yao inserts the needles and most don't hurt. There are few that are painful, fortunately, after a few minutes, the pain subsides. Yao explains the painful areas are where the *chi* is blocked. I have absolutely no idea what she's talking about; again, I figure, in time, I will understand.

She puts in one acupuncture needle at the crown of my head, explaining it's for the TBI and it will help. I don't know if it's true or not, but again, what have I got to lose. After all the needles are in, she rolls an herb called mugwort into a very small ball. Next, she places the herb on top of a few needles and lights the herb. This technique is called moxibustion and supposedly it helps to open an acupuncture point and area. The herb smolders and the warmth feels really good as it flows through the needles and into my body. Yao tells me to relax and let the needles do their work. Quickly, I fall asleep.

Forty-five minutes later, Yao quietly opens the door carrying two plastic grocery bags. Inside are twelve individual-wrapped paper bags filled with herbs, which she calls my prescription. I need to soak and cook three bags of herbs and drink my herbal tea: three days on and four days off. This *tea* is the worst stuff I've ever tasted; it's like drinking watered down dirt with an extremely nasty, bitter after taste. Now I know why medicine tastes so bad, it's so people get healthy as quickly as possible so they don't have to take this foul medicine. Though I don't like the tea, acupuncture is very intriguing and I sense there's much to experience.

9

CROSSROADS
AND A NEW
PATHWAY
AUGUST 1993

Rising within me is a tremendous drive to resume my brain healing journey, but the effects from the cancer, the treatments, and the intense grief are still overwhelming. Instead of focusing on what I can't do, I decide to open up and focus on what I can do. On a warm summer afternoon, I take a deep breath and pray again for help and direction in my brain healing journey. *This time, I am all in; I have completely surrendered. Intentionally, I quiet my mind in order to be open, listen, and receive.* Immediately, I have a gut sense that martial arts will help. At first, I'm surprised by the clarity, precision, and swiftness with which the answer came. I smile. Before I prayed, I had wholeheartedly surrendered – as I do in my daily surrender to stay sober. Previously, I thought I was humble, open to receive, and had surrendered when I asked for help for my next right step in my brain healing journey, but *now* I know I am.

Before I got sober, I did martial arts for about a year. I was astonished how much more I was able to do and achieve than I thought I could. I loved martial arts, but I didn't stick with it because the drinking had full control of me.

My powerful past reminds me that possibilities are endless and limitations are only in the mind, but not in mine. Enthusiastically, I grab the phone book and call martial art schools in the area. I'm looking for an art that focuses on health, discipline, longevity, and of course, self-defense. I need to be positively challenged – mentally and physically. After much research I choose to study the art of Kung Fu. **In time, I'll realize the particular martial art, school, or teacher chosen has no bearing in my brain healing journey. No one in the world knows how to completely heal the brain; therefore, no one can guide me. The responsibility for discovering a solution to the TBI rests squarely on my shoulders.**

A REFRESHING CHANGE EARLY SEPTEMBER 1993

Opening the door to the martial art school, I see students powerfully and gracefully moving through forms. Their memory and physical abilities are impressive; *this is how I want to be!* Before crossing the threshold, I bow as a sign of respect and take a moment to leave any problems of the day and life behind. This is my time to train and have fun. Wow, what a concept – having fun while learning and working out. Way cool!

I put my shoes and small duffle bag in the storage area, and before entering the training area, I bow again. Walking barefoot feels weird and good at the same time; I don't walk around barefoot at home. I'm wearing a favorite t-shirt and sweat pants, which helps me feel a little more comfortable. I'm also still using my constant companions: earplugs, dark glasses, and extra sturdy wrist brace. The latest news about my wrist is there's no hope for improvement: it needs to be surgically frozen in one position to relieve the massive pain. I'm not keen on the idea of surgery and decide to keep working on getting my normal range of motion; I believe it's about 30 more degrees.

I look around the school trying to figure out what I'm supposed to do and where to go. I feel lost like I'm the new kid at school. *Oh yea, I am the new kid at school*! Inside, I laugh at myself while trying to look cool on the outside. The gong is rung and I line up with the other white belts. Class begins with a bow and a very brief meditation in the kneeling position, which I'm unable to do. Instead, I sit on the floor with my legs crossed. The warm-ups begin with simple exercises: push-ups, sit-ups, squats, leg lifts, and all sort of stretching. The Cat Style push-ups look like a cat stretching its spine in both directions. But, I can barely do one-tenth of the exercises. I'm not able to do a single push up on my knees, and when I stretch I can only gaze at my feet. I'm in worse shape than I thought. That's okay; it's not the hare that wins the race, I'll be the turtle, slow and steadfast.

Later, two very kind Black Belts graciously teach me the correct kneeling position; the weight is shifted forward off the ankles. Though I'm unable to do the posture, they reassure me that with time and effort, I will improve, and one day, I will be able to do it. They move on to help other students, and I realize they just said, "One day, you will be able to do the kneeling posture." Hold the presses – someone said I will be able to do something! What a refreshing change from all the pessimistic "no's and never's" and "impossible's!"

10

AN INSIGHT INTO
MY BRAIN
HEALING
JOURNEY

To help me understand the overall method of martial arts, I utilize my experience of re-learning how to write after the TBI. Writing a word is the basic stances, strikes, and kicks, and connecting the movements are called forms.

My beginner's group is very quickly taught the basic stances and strikes, then moves on to a form. But, I'm struggling with the basic stances, never mind all the different strikes. I have a gut sense to continue moving forward with the group instead of getting left behind. At home, I'll work on the basics and everything else.

A few minutes pass and I am so glad I kept moving forward. There's one set of simple movements, which are absolutely fascinating: *simultaneously* blocking, punching, and kicking. [To watch this video go to my website www.brainphoenix.com and look for Chapter link, video is also on YouTube.] I keep working at getting, or as I like to say, *owning* these simple simultaneous opposite movements, but no matter how much I try, they're still baffling. As the doubts try to set up housekeeping, I look up and see my fellow students, all with intact brains, looking just as confused as I feel. Beside me, two students are quietly talking, "Before I began studying martial arts I thought I knew the difference between my rights and lefts." "Yea, me too, but when you add on arms and legs, it's like learning a whole other language." I am beyond relieved; my busted brain is getting in the way, but it's not all TBI. Rather than feed the doubts, I figure my best approach is to simplify everything.

I continue working out, and although some students have stopped coming to class. The students who are still training from my beginner's group, the next beginner's group, and the next have tested up one or two belt levels. Yet, I'm still a white belt. It's very easy to see their improvements physically and mentally. Even their self-confidence has blossomed as they go about their business of working out and living life.

Once again, I've run smack into the wall of TBI. I take a deep breath, and notice my aching heart and chest closing to protect it. If I give up now, I'll never, ever discover a solution to TBI, and I will quit everything that gets tough. I ask myself a question. How badly do I want to be completely free of this TBI, be reconnected, and to what lengths will I go? In the past, this question and questions similar to this have always helped change my mind-set and kept me persevering.

I take another deep breath and decide to open and surrender in a good way: *I am all in – my actions will speak louder than words.* Immediately, I get a huge gut sense; if I can own these simple, simultaneous opposite movements, *my brain can do anything. I can do anything.* I need to be aware of how my muscles, joints, etc. are moving, working, and connecting while simultaneously blocking, striking, and kicking. Just as important, I don't need to be concerned with how the outer movements look. I decide to trust my gut; again, it would be foolish not to.

With enthusiasm, I'm aware of my muscles, joints, etc. and how they're moving while I'm simultaneously blocking and punching. After a few minutes, something unexpected happens. I experience a *push-pull* within my brain; I'm aware of both sides of my brain by simultaneously working opposite sides of my body. For the first time since the TBI, there's a smidgen of stirring in my brain, *more precisely inside the thick, blurry glass wall*! It's like my brain is catching the first sniff of hot coffee while snuggled in a warm bed on a cold winter morning. But, my brain isn't ready to wake up. In my brain, there are many connections which are off, creating many misses physically and mentally. Although I don't know how to unite these brain connections, my gut sense is that in time, I'll figure it out. *Next, I get a gut sense that this slight brain awakening is a gift encouraging me to keep persevering and nothing more.* Without any rational reason to trust, I decide I'm all in. I will trust what I'm led to do, and I will do all the work to get all the results. As soon as I make the decision, I get the biggest gut sense ever.

There isn't a person or organization in the world that has the tools or the knowledge to free me from the prison in my brain. Nothing and no one from the outside can liberate me. The solution is *inside* me. I need to learn the basic tools, information, and principles of martial arts, acupuncture, and other methods; then, I need to transform these basic tools into new positive, healthy brain healing techniques. *My number one brain healing technique will be to continue delving deeper into my inner awareness training; being aware of how my inner body moves, connects, works, and responds.*

Also, intellectual outside techniques and knowledge of anatomy and how the body works are *not* the solution. My inner awareness training *needs* to be experienced. I must simplify everything so I can continue delving deeper into my inner awareness training.

In addition, every step and technique needs to become second nature before moving onto the next level. This means I need to get to the point where I no longer have to consciously think and focus on what I'm doing to develop my inner awareness; yet, it's easy and natural to be aware and stay aware of what's occurring within my inner body.

My laboratory will be my body, and I'll measure my progress based on results. Does my speech, memory, and energy level improve and by how much? Am I able to tolerate noise and light, and by how much? Or am I stagnating? *Of the utmost importance is to always delve deeper into my inner awareness training. Again, my outside progress and achievements must not be the focus; they will only take me off course.*

Missteps and techniques that don't work are a natural part of any journey. Learn from them, they may lead to great breakthroughs. Though it's important to figure out why a technique didn't work; a dead-end path, it's crucial not to get stuck on the why's. Spending too much time on why something didn't work could take my brain healing journey off course. Accept when a path dead-ends and keep moving forward.

Be relentless, my brain healing journey is uncharted territory. Always keep delving deeper into my inner awareness training with everything I do. Always keep improving on what works. With this mind-set I will naturally be led to my next right step. Have faith and trust – I will discover a way to completely heal and enhance my brain better than before the TBI. Always remember, be relentless, the solution is inside me.

My gut sense concludes, and for the first time I have real hope inside the prison in my brain. One day, I will liberate and reconnect myself and be better than before the TBI. Although I don't have scientific facts or evidence to back this up, and in many ways it doesn't make sense. I will not discount or second guess an insight like I did before the accident – that would be nuts. I take a deep breath and become aware of my inner body; how the muscles, joints, etc. are moving as I simultaneously block, punch, and kick.

PHASE 1

STEP BY STEP
DELVING DEEPER
INTO
MY INNER
AWARENESS
TRAINING

11

SIMULTANEOUSLY STRENGTHENING MY BODY WHILE CHALLENGING MY BRAIN LATE SEPTEMBER 1993

*The next five months are power packed with enormous progress and outstanding discoveries – a direct result of my #1 brain healing technique – my inner awareness training. I've chosen to write these extraordinary experiences into the next three chapters with the hope of making it clearer. Again, keep in mind that all of my improvements are happening simultaneously.

I focus on my hands and feet while simultaneously blocking, punching, and kicking. While blocking my face, I brush my nose and startle myself. I look around. I'm alone at home, no one can see me, yet I'm embarrassed. I take a breath, and simplify my practice to only simultaneously blocking and punching. Although I practice diligently, I'm getting nowhere. The frustrations and doubts – fears start gnawing at me. In my head, I hear a favorite saying of one of my mentors, "Keep your eye on the ball." I change my perspective.

The answer is inside me. Focusing on the outer movements is another external method, which will always fail. The key to all my success has been to always delve deeper into my inner awareness training. The solution is inside me!

I decide to coach myself, in order to do everything I can to motivate me. Encouragingly I say, "It's easy to be aware of my inner body. C'mon Cath, you can do it; do what has always worked. *Keep delving deeper into my precious inner awareness training.*" Although it feels a little weird coaching myself out loud, it inspires me.

I begin again; *first* I'm aware and stay aware of my inner body; *then*, I simultaneously block and strike. Little by little, I'm aware of the muscles, joints, etc. moving in my right upper arm. The inner movements are different than picking up a backpack or pen, and writing. Next, I delve deeper into my inner awareness by being aware of my left shoulder joint; the ball is rotating in the socket as I pull my elbow back. Simultaneously, I'm aware of my right upper inner arm. Discovering more of the inner world inside my body is extraordinary. [To watch the related video go to my website www.brainphoenix.com and look for Chapter links, video is also on YouTube. This is the last video. Although some people may want more videos of techniques of my Brain

Phoenix ™ method; videos are inadequate. My method must be taught in person.]

With childlike wonder, I become immersed with the inner movements; I'm aware of the push – pull of muscles, joints, etc. in both arms as I simultaneously block and punch. I am stunned at how simple, easy, and fun it is to be aware of my inner body. *When it's completely natural to be aware of my inner body while simultaneously blocking and striking, it's time to move to my next right step; adding new strikes and kicks.* Simultaneously, I'm also expanding my inner awareness training by reaching for and grasping everyday objects; fork, spoon, knife, cup, food, door knob, keys, and leash to name a few. Again, my focus must first be on delving deeper into my inner awareness training, not on the outside techniques and success.

In addition, the years of being absolutely dependent on earplugs and dark sunglasses have finally helped me in ways I couldn't have imagined. It's completely natural to be aware of how my breathing and heart beat changes doing my brain healing training while walking, hiking, and sitting in a comfortable chair. Also, I'm already aware of the difference in sounds and sensations of drinking water, a chocolate milk shake, or eating various foods. What I and others saw as an unfortunate necessity, ear plugs and dark sunglasses, have been transformed into an asset. *Out of every negative have come many positive, healthy experiences and transformations because I've learned to be open, to look for, and to purposefully work for them.*

I've been with my body 24/7 from the moment I was born, but I hadn't really paid attention to how my inner body moves, connects, works, and responds – until I began developing my precious inner awareness training. What little I knew about the human body, I learned in biology class. On the other hand, I now realize that I've been aware of my inner body my entire life: when I needed to rest, eat, go to the bathroom, and so on. I've been developing my inner awareness since I was a small child.

By step by step delving deeper into my inner awareness training, it is improving by leaps and bounds. But, there's only miniscule progress with the outer movements; they still suck. Hidden within this obstacle is another great gift. Even though I'm not doing the simultaneous movements correctly, it's very easy and natural to delve deeper into my precious inner awareness training, and the benefits are: a slight increase with my outer focus; including when I do the external movements, and there is a tiny improvement in my energy level. I believe I've found another path to improve my inner awareness training. Though I still don't understand why everything isn't improving at the same rate, out loud I tell myself. *"Don't focus on how the outer movements look or the three-tiered progress – keep delving deeper into my inner awareness training – no matter what."*

Next, I have gut sense to slow down the outer simultaneous movements. Even though this seems backwards, my inner awareness improves. It's much easier to be aware of my muscles, bones, and joints etc. in my fists, arms, shoulders, and upper chest. But, there's a huge hitch with my right shoulder, wrist, and other parts of my body that were injured in the accident. My first thought is bummer, until I realize this is another great gift. *Being aware of the differences and similarities between the healthy and damaged areas is improving my inner awareness.* I'm also a little more mindful. First, with the inner movements; then, the outer movements while blocking, punching, and kicking, and also cooking food, writing notes for the forms, walking, and hiking with Maja, etc. *My precious inner awareness training is the gift that keeps on giving.*

REGAINING MY FOOTING

While I delve deeper into my precious inner awareness training with the: simultaneous opposite movements, using everyday objects, and doing daily activities, *I am simultaneously working on being aware of my feet*. My hope is to reconnect with my feet. I begin by intensely watching my bare feet as they gently nestle into the medium thick rug. Slowly, I pivot one foot outward softly over the surface and return it to its natural position then the other foot. A shiver runs up my spine. I can see my bare feet, but my brain still isn't able to find my feet or the rug; it's like my feet have been severed from my body. Why am I still surprised by a disconnection that's outside the prison in my brain?

I take a breath and slowly exhale. Calmly, I shake my body and stretch my neck side to side. I wiggle my toes and slightly grasp the rug until my feet are snuggled into the carpet. I stare at my feet while slowly pivoting one foot then the other, repeating my experiment over and over again.

The sparrows squabbling in the apple tree distract me. I look out the window and wonder, why do sparrows fight so much? As soon as the thought finishes, my entertainment flies off. Next, I notice the noise coming from the electronic devices in the room, which are off. A few moments later, I remember I'm trying to do my brain healing training. I start giving myself a hard time for losing focus, but kicking my butt is a waste of precious energy and being critical will only take me off-course. I need to be wise with my words and energy. I also know that when I enjoy what

I'm doing, I make more progress. I decide that whenever I get distracted, I'll gently say; "That's ok. Re-focus, do your best, and have fun!"

I continue watching my feet as they move over the carpet, but I'm not making progress, I'm just getting aggravated. I remember what Dad told me, "Cathy, calm down, it's not going help getting frustrated. Relax, calm down." I ask myself a question, "How badly do I want to be free of the TBI and be reconnected? My question changes my mind-set and puts me back on track. I decide to use my *entire* body to focus inside, not just my eyes and ears. Immediately, I have a huge gut sense; *watching my feet is an external method, which will always fail – the solution is inside me.*

Why do I keep focusing on the outer movements? Is it because that's what I've always been taught in sports, work, and hobbies? Probably, but that doesn't matter anymore because focusing on the outer movements is not working, and my precious inner awareness training is working phenomenally well!

I begin again. *First, I'm aware and stay aware of my inner body: how my muscles, joints, etc. are moving, connecting, and working.* Slowly, I safely pivot one foot softly over the rug and return it to its natural position then the other foot, *without looking at my feet.* After a few minutes I'm astounded; I'm slightly aware of the muscles, small bones, and joints etc. moving *inside* my feet. Also, I'm now aware that my left foot feels warmer from the sunlight streaming through the east window. Eagerly, I continue and become aware of a little bit of sweat building up on my feet, especially my left foot. My toes are slightly getting stuck as they move over the carpet and things feel tight inside my feet then they release as the movements continue. *This is a new inner awareness! I feel like a hound dog that's caught the scent, and the trail is inside me!*

I grip the rug with my toes, then relax; I get goose bumps – chicken skin kine all over. Being aware of muscles, joints, etc. tightening and releasing is invigorating – it's like I've got *feelers inside my body.* When I finish my brain healing training, I still my movements and sink into the carpet. I step away and notice the impression of my feet in the rug. My right foot is clearly marked, but the impression of my left foot is quickly disappearing into the carpet. Huh, I didn't know most of my weight was on my right side; I thought I was balanced. Bummer, another thing to work on. No, this is another great gift! If I don't know something is wrong, how can I fix it? I go back to the saying; figure out the problem, and it will be easier to find then apply the solution. By discovering the problem, I don't have to keep making the same mistake over and over again.

To improve my inner awareness, I decide to simultaneously be aware of my inner feet and distributing my weight equally while pivoting each foot over the rug. *At first it seems like a lot to handle; however, by paying attention to what is happening inside my body, it rather quickly becomes natural, and I experience the biggest improvement in my inner awareness training. It is enormously easy to be aware of how my inner body is moving, connecting, and working. Simultaneously being aware of doing two techniques has immensely helped to delve deeper into my inner awareness training.*

When it's completely natural to be aware of my inner feet and weight distribution, I'm ready to move on. However, my balance and weight distribution are far from perfect and I'm not sure why. I have a gut sense that there's more to balance, and in time, the pieces will come together.

Next, I add on another task – simultaneously being aware of my inner body while blocking, striking, and kicking, and also balancing or distributing my weight equally. *I am aware of the flow in the muscles, bones, and joints, etc. in my hands, arms, chest, shoulders, and inner feet, yet I don't have to consciously focus on being aware. I am shocked; simultaneously doing more techniques is helping me to be a little more aware of the inner movements, and I am a little clearer.* I continue practicing, and once again, it's time to move forward when I 100% own my number one technique, my inner awareness training, while doing these outer movements. I remind myself that it's not important how my outer movements look and that my balance is far from perfect; it's ALL about delving deeper into my inner awareness training.

Encouraged by my success, I step up my inner awareness training by being aware of my inner feet and body while standing barefoot on numerous surfaces in and around my home: carpet, tile, hardwood and parquet floors, slate, grass, dirt, wood decking, concrete, and anything else I can find. Of course, I'm simultaneously working on being aware of my balance too. With each new surface I'm aware of the slight changes in my muscles, joints, etc. There is also a small improvement in my outer focus in the foreign outside world and a slight increase in my energy level. Again, my progress is occurring from the inside out (always my inner awareness first) and it's still happening at the same three-tiered rate.

Next, I purposefully walk, one step at a time, on the different surfaces. After that, I practice on each surface: stepping, turning, and blocking, the simultaneous opposite movements, and ALL my other techniques, which improve my inner awareness little by little. I'm also enjoying taking Maja for longer walks and hikes, which is a great opportunity to practice my inner awareness training while wearing sneakers and boots. Though wearing footwear is not as good as being barefoot, it's easy to be naturally aware of my inner feet and body while traversing: gravel, asphalt, mud, dirt, rocks, hills, and steep terrain. Another benefit from my inner awareness training is that I'm a little more present, clearer, and aware of the foreign outside world. I take great joy in spotting birds, deer, coyote, other animals, their tracks and feathers, and also flowers. I sense my inner awareness training is helping me tap into my natural healthy state.

Although I am very happy with the progress, I know I need to have solid footing to be successful in my brain healing journey. My next right step is rooting training, or sinking my energy into the earth, which I don't believe in. Supposedly, rooting enhances balance and other things. My bare feet grasp the ground, and I'm aware of my muscles and body getting tense. My precious energy is also being drained. I'm definitely not getting the concept of rooting. The straining reminds me of when I'm constipated and trying to poop. Shortly thereafter, I realize it's the *mind or visualization* that does most of the work to root, not the muscles. I laugh at myself and how funny I must have looked with a scrunched up face.

I decide to change my approach to rooting by using the simple concept of visualization which athletes, martial artists, and Olympians successfully use. I visualize myself as a massive tree with life giving energy flowing through my head, into my neck, up my arms and into my trunk, legs, and feet, then entering the ground as my roots reach deep and purposefully into the earth. Next, I envision the vibrant energy rising through my strong and hearty root system into my feet, legs, trunk, then branching into my arms, hands, and head. Even though I don't feel rooted and energy moving in me, I've made an *enormous transformation and a mammoth advancement in my inner awareness training. I am simultaneously aware of the flow of numerous muscles, joints, etc., rather than individual parts. Step by step, I love that I continue making great progress in my brain healing journey; it's simple, easy, and a whole lot of fun blazing this trail.*

IT'S EASY WORKING SMARTER NOT HARDER

Around the time I started at the martial art school, I began volunteering at a local horse riding center for people with disabilities. Although I qualify to be a client and ride the horses, I choose to volunteer because I've received so much help since the TBI; it's time to give back.

I love being around the horses; they make my heart sing, and there's a wonderful, palpable spirit at the riding center. The staff is encouraging, respectful, and helpful, and they want everyone to succeed. It is refreshing to be around people whose actions speak louder than their words.

I'm doing two jobs at the riding center: mucking out the stalls and horse leader. Mucking out the stalls is an early morning task which I do once a week. It's pretty simple: raking and shoveling the horse poop into a wheel barrel and dumping the contents into a big pile in the middle of the field. I thought my wrist might give me trouble, but like the rest of my body, my wrist is getting a little stronger and more flexible. I take pride in making a clean, safe place for the horses to live. I also thoroughly enjoy watching the horses' ears perk up when they see me, because they know I always carry special treats.

My job as a horse leader is extensive and a great responsibility.

First, I do an overall check-up of the horse, making sure the horse is physically and mentally ready to do a class. Next, I groom the horse: picking the hooves, brushing the coat, combing the mane, and putting on the blanket, saddle, bit and reins. During class, I need to be in control of my horse while focusing on the rider and the two volunteers on either side of the horse. I also need to be aware of the other horses, their riders, their volunteers, and the entire ring area. I must do all of these activities while watching and following the teacher's instructions.

Today is my first time as a horse leader and I'm a little nervous. While preparing the horse, I become aware that my chest and shoulders are tight and that my abdomen is in a knot. My shoulders slump; I'm not sure I can be a horse leader – it is a major responsibility. I step back from the horse. If I don't change my mind-set, the horse will pick up on my negative energy; doubts – fear, and he'll make my job enormously more challenging. Consciously, I focus to my inner body, and immediately, I'm aware of my muscles, joints, etc. and how they're moving, connecting, and working. I love that focusing on my inner awareness training calms and centers me. I take a deep, slow breath and return to preparing the horse.

While brushing the horse's coat, I have *a huge gut sense. I need to intentionally do my inner awareness training the **entire time** I'm doing my job as a horse leader, or I will completely flounder.* Consciously, I deepen my inner awareness, becoming aware of how my muscles, joints, etc. are moving, connecting, and working while I finish preparing the horse, and walking him to the covered area next to the barn. During class, I'm pleasantly surprised how easy it is to naturally deepen my inner awareness to a whole new level; I'm simultaneously aware of new and previous areas of my inner body. *Inside, it feels like I'm getting in sync with the horse.* Though I'm not sure what this in sync thing is, I am definitely moving in the right direction.

After class, the instructor compliments me on doing a great job. I'm relieved and very happy. However, my energy is drained and I'm not able to do my inner awareness training. I return home, sleep for hours, yet wake up exhausted. The next three days my ability to do my brain healing training is greatly diminished. Although I continue doing a great job as a horse leader, after each class my inner awareness and energy are depleted. It's obvious, rest and putting in more time and effort as a horse leader is not the answer.

At the same time, I've hit another wall – there's only so much inner awareness I can develop with the basic simultaneous opposite movements: block, punch, kick, and rooting. To ascend to the next level of my inner awareness training, *I need to continually change how I move my body in order to become aware of new muscles, joints, etc.* This means I need to remember, longer and more complex forms, but I am incapable of remembering new movements and forms. Dejavu; it's my university experience all over again.

Since the accident, I've relied on people with intact brains for memory – this is a dead-end path. First, there's no one to ask while doing my brain healing training. Second, and more importantly, relying on others for memory is a powerless, negative pattern which will not help me in my brain healing journey. If I don't overcome these massive obstacles, I will not be able to continue honing my phenomenal inner awareness, and I'll never discover a way out of this TBI. I need to find a solution.

I recall an event that occurred when I started at the riding center; I remember it like it was happening right now. On a bright, cold, windy autumn morning, I tug my old cowboy hat down, zip up my coat, and walk toward the stable. I put the halter on the horse, walk through the gate and close it; then, brace myself for the blustery west wind. We enter an open area and a huge gust of wind whips up the dirt stinging my eyes and spooking the horse. The horse rears up; his front legs are thrashing in the air. I struggle to control the horse, but I'm no match for this powerful animal. My heart is pounding; it feels like it's going to explode out my chest. I don't know what to do.

A farrier, a person who shoes horses, walks over and quietly asks if he can help; his energy is calm and centered. I've never seen this man before, and with all the commotion going on, all I can do is nod my head up and down. He takes the rope and walks the horse in a small circle. Immediately, the horse calms down. When the horse acts up, he gives a quick yank on the rope and the horse follows his command. This man is a miracle worker!

The farrier hands back the rope while looking deeply into my eyes. He turns and walks toward the forge next to his truck. He's about halfway to the forge when the horse rears up again. Calmly, he returns and in a quiet manner asks, "Do you want to learn how to handle a horse?" Without hesitating I say, "Yes!"

He teaches me the basics: how to hold the rope and to not loop the rope around my hand in case the horse decides to take off. He jokes that it's good to have your fingers and arm attached to your body and not to the horse. He demonstrates how to lead a horse making sure there's enough space for the horse and handler to clear a gate, and to always close a gate after opening it. Next, he shows me how to lead a horse in a small circle as soon as a horse acts up or gives attitude. With each instruction, I demonstrate what he's shown before we move on to the next lesson. In a matter of a few minutes, I own the very basics of how to handle a horse.

I look the farrier squarely in the eye, thank him for all his help, and ask if he has any other suggestions. My powerful past has taught me to ask for suggestions from people who are experienced, knowledgeable, and centered. On the other hand, I've learned to take with a grain of salt people who give advice, opinions, and suggestions without being asked, especially when they don't have any responsibility in the situation.

With one finger, the farrier raises his hat, turns his head to the side, leans in, and looks me squarely in the eye. He's sizing me up. When he's satisfied that I really want to learn, he shares these words of wisdom which I will treasure for the rest of my life.

"If you think a horse can do something then most likely the horse will do it. But, if you don't think a horse can do something then most likely he won't."

He leans in closer, making sure I understand. When he's

satisfied, he walks back to his forge and continues shoeing a horse.

I tie my horse to the hitching post and think about his words of wisdom while preparing the horse for class. I'm also watching how the farrier interacts with the staff, other people, and horses. He's a quiet, humble man; it's easy to sense and see that he's comfortable with who he is and what he does. At the time I didn't know that was the first and last time I'd see that farrier.

The next three days I pondered his words. In an instant, they transform into a big, power packed phrase – technique. *If I say, It's Easy to do a task and continue positively thinking and speaking while consistently taking healthy actions – most likely it will be easier, no matter how many people say it's impossible or difficult to do. On the other hand, if I keep thinking and speaking pessimistically about how hard or impossible something is to do and consistently take negative actions – most likely it will be even harder or impossible to do.*

I decide to implement the positive mind-set of *It's Easy* into my brain healing journey and life. *It's Easy* to do my job as a volunteer horse leader, and afterwards, I will have more energy for my inner awareness and brain healing training. *It's Easy* to *always* delve deeper into my inner awareness training which will help me develop a method to remember longer, more complex martial art forms and information. *IT'S EASY to discover a solution to TBI!*

Before the next class at the riding center, I reflect on my recent experiences with horses. It's almost effortless to deepen my inner awareness when I'm around horses. Is it because horses are naturally aware from the inside out? Horses do seem to be innately aware of people, animals, and situations; they are always present, in the now. Hmm, could I learn from horses how to improve my inner awareness training? Immediately, I get a huge gut sense – horses will help me delve deeper into a whole new level of inner awareness and connections within my body. Rather than do any more mental gymnastics, I decide to trust my gut; again, it would be nuts not to.

The next class, I arrive earlier and prepare the horse. I walk the horse to a quiet area and face him while calmly saying to myself, *It's Easy* to deepen my inner awareness. Purposefully, I'm aware of my inner body. In a matter of seconds, my inner awareness naturally deepens; I'm aware and making connections inside my body; muscles, joints, etc., to a whole, new deeper level while I'm simultaneously aware of the horse. I realize every inner awareness discovery before was at a superficial or pre-school level. To be clear, this isn't bonding with the horse and it's much more than being aware of my muscles, joints, etc. There are no words to adequately describe what I'm experiencing. The best way to explain this is I've reached a new innate level of inner awareness. But, describing my experience with words is like trying to explain how a delicious hot apple pie tastes to someone who's never had dessert. Again, words are paltry – *my inner awareness training needs to be personally experienced. In the future, I will need to teach my brain healing method in person; reading about it or listening to me talking about my method would be totally inadequate.*

I continue deepening my inner awareness with different horses. To my surprise, after working with a few horses, I don't have to face the horse to consciously develop new and deeper levels of inner awareness. To be clear my inner awareness and connections occur first, within myself, then with the horses. What's interesting is each horse has a slightly different way of being inwardly aware and connected; and it's my job to adapt to them. After working with eight horses, it's completely natural to be aware and connected to my inner body, from the inside out, while also being aware and having an inner connection with each horse.

For the first time since the TBI, it's easy to be aware and connected with another being. The benefits from my inner awareness training are beyond exceptional. I am a little clearer, several layers of fog have lifted, and I have more energy. I am delighted how easy it is to perform all my tasks as a horse leader and do them well. I'm also doing my brain healing training for longer periods of time, and finish with even more inner awareness and energy.

I'm also taking Maja the wonder pup for longer hikes. However, some evenings I don't have the energy to go to my martial art class, which tells me I need to continue delving deeper into my precious inner awareness training.

After working with a few more horses, I realize that I do not need to be around a horse to discover new and deeper levels of inner awareness and connections. This is beyond cool; I don't need a horse, a person, or anything outside of me to improve my inner awareness – *the solution is inside me*!

While I'm discovering new levels of inner awareness and connections – I am simultaneously developing a method to help me remember longer and more complex martial art forms and information. In time, I will call this My Simultaneous Brain Learning Method. As always, the sole purpose of every technique in my brain healing journey is to continue delving deeper into my precious inner awareness training.

First, I *decide* to go back to an old reliable tool, my tape recorder, to write notes for the martial art forms. I record a section of a form, speaking the same words other people use to describe the movements. Returning home, my excitement grows as I look for a notebook and pen. At the kitchen table, I rewind the audio tape, press play, and quickly notice a major problem. In frustration, I yell at the tape, "Turn where? What kind of stance? Do this. What does do this mean?" Arghh, I've picked up the bad habit of being vague with my words.

Rather than persevere backwards, I change my mind-set by *making a decision*. I will train myself to *precisely think, speak, and write* each martial art movement and form as if I'm teaching a blind person or a person like me with a busted brain. Although this is a gargantuan, super-human task, considering the vast majority of brain damage is in my left temporal lobe – the verbal center. I will have faith in me and my brain healing training; I will succeed – *It's Easy*!

I stand up on the parquet floor, and this time I'm aware of my inner body which relaxes me. I smile. I love being aware of my muscles, joints, etc. in my: fingers, hands, arms, shoulders, chest, and inner feet. I press the audio record button, and as a sign of respect I bow before beginning the form. I speak into the tape recorder; "Bow north." I step forward, and I'm slightly aware of the muscles warming up in my upper forward leg. However, I am still surprised at how challenging it is to be aware of muscles, joints, etc. that are further away from the prison in my brain.

The muscles in my upper, forward leg feel like they're on fire, which makes it a little easier to be aware that I'm in a right bow stance. I speak into the tape recorder; "Right bow stance north." Next, I simultaneous block and strike while holding the tape recorder. Thankfully, the tape recorder has a wrist strap. Move by move, I first become aware of how the muscles, joints, etc. are moving and connecting; then, I'm able to record each movement to the best of my ability. I finish *physically* doing the form and recording the movements in my tape recorder. I really want to *write* my notes, but I'm too tired and take a nap. Later, I carefully *listen* to the audio tape and *write* my notes as clearly and precisely as I can. Next, I *read* my notes to get the information deeper into my brain. *Unknowingly*, as I'm listening, writing, and reading my notes, I'm SIMULTANEOUSLY aware of my inner body, and I'm also speaking the words *out loud* with the same tempo and tone as I recorded them.

I place my notes and pen in my back waistband. While I'm *physically* doing the form, I'm aware of how my muscles, joints, etc. are moving and connecting. I'm also unknowingly speaking the movements out loud with the same tempo and tone as I recorded, listened, wrote, and read them. When I forget a move, especially a pesky transitional move, which are quite challenging for people with intact brains, I check my notes. The majority of time my notes are incorrect or not precise enough. Quickly, I fix my notes and continue physically doing the form. With each new movement and form I do, I become aware of new muscles, joints, and areas of my inner body. Again, I wonder if I should I learn the names of the different parts of my inner body? No, the outside intellectual knowledge and focus will take me off-course. Focus on delving deeper into my inner awareness training!

To make sure my notes are correct, I practice the forms with my new workout buddies at school and during class. I continue *re-writing* and clarifying my notes as precisely as I can. In addition, I stop using the tape recorder when I'm confident my notes are correct; I don't want to rely on any outside technique or tool which would take me off-course.

Rather quickly, it becomes a little more natural to do my inner awareness training while doing all the new movements, which means I don't have to consciously focus on being aware of my muscles, joints, etc. and how they move and connect, yet I am still aware of *ALL* of them. My memory, verbal and writing skills, and energy level have slightly improved. *On my own I am doing my forms, and I own more forms, without relying on my notes, an outside tool. In my gut, I get a very strong sense – my brain has been waiting for me to delve deeper into my precious inner awareness training.*

Next, I practice my forms on different surfaces: rugs, slate, wood deck, and grass, etc. I wonder, if I simultaneously apply more techniques will that deepen my inner awareness and help me discover solutions to fatigue and other obstacles? Well, if I had more energy, I could do my brain healing training longer. Though I have to be careful; I have a tendency to push myself too hard, especially when I'm around people with intact brains. One martial art class takes about 2 ½ days to recover from; however, I believe the majority of fatigue is from the radiation treatments and grief. On the other hand, trying to find a balance in how much to do my brain healing training, volunteering, martial art classes, and daily activities – *all* of which are helping to improve my inner awareness is – a very interesting quandary. I believe if I had an intact brain, it would be a huge challenge to find a balance. In my gut, I get another very strong sense to keep persevering with *everything*.

I *decide* to turn my downtime into a positive by integrating the tool of *visualization*, which I utilize in my rooting training. In a quiet room at home, I sit with my eyes closed. First, I become aware of my muscles, joints, etc. Next, I visualize myself doing each movement in a form. Without realizing it, at times, I'm simultaneously speaking the movements out loud and moving my arms and legs a bit. When I forget a move, I check my notes. Again, most times, my notes aren't clear enough. As I'm fixing my notes, I notice there are more details and fewer mistakes with my newer notes for forms than with the older notes and I'm not sure why.

Move by move, I envision myself performing each form which naturally deepens my inner awareness. In my minds-eye, I see my stances deepening, I'm striking with accuracy and power, and of course, I'm having a blast. When I'm physically able to train again, I experience major improvements with my inner awareness training; though, there are only slight improvements with my memory, verbal, and physical skills.

Visualizing forms quickly becomes second nature. Next, I make it a game or play to visualize my notes. In time, I will, step by step, improve my visualization of my notes: what page a single movement from a form is on, precisely where a movement is on a page; then, I will visualize my forms and notes in more lively environments and while doing daily activities. Although visualization and watching students do forms ingrains the forms deeper into me, *visualization does not take the place of physically doing forms to delve deeper into my inner awareness. Again, relying on outside techniques and people is not a solution.*

The next technique I simultaneously apply is learning Chinese words and phrases that describe the movements and forms. Learning a *new language skill* is quite hilarious. Not only is my Chinese accent horrible, most of the time I need a language interpreter for my New Englandese, never mind another language! Literally, I've had to change the word "car" to "vehicle" because no one in Colorado can understand me. I take in stride the good-natured ribbing about my accent from my workout buddies and others. In addition, my verbal skills are receiving a boost by learning new definitions for English words like sweeping. For example, sweeping a broom, and in martial arts, there are many techniques for sweeping a person's leg.

I'm also experiencing a very unexpected and amusing development with my new language skill. Other students, with intact brains, are asking me how to say Chinese words and phrases. The first few times this happened, I was shocked and thought – Who's the one with a TBI? Then, I smile from ear to ear, take a deep breath, and speak the Chinese word or phrase. Before returning to do my forms, I tell each person to ask someone who has a better grasp of the Chinese language for the correct pronunciation. To my surprise and delight, more and more students, all with intact brains, continue to ask me how to correctly say Chinese words and phrases. It is also very humorous listening to people arguing about the correct pronunciation of a Chinese word when they don't have a clue how to speak Chinese. Some people try to get me to weigh in on the correct spelling and pronunciation of Chinese words and phrases. But, I do not care – this is an outside focus which will only pull me off-course.

Simultaneously, I'm implementing other techniques that I've been utilizing for a long time: *consistently making healthy decisions, taking positive actions, learning from successes and missteps and cleaning up my missteps, having fun, being enthusiastic, and enjoying each moment while working diligently.* Again, in time, I will call this my Simultaneous Brain Learning Method; ten techniques and counting because I'm always looking to improve on what works.

My Simultaneous Brain Learning Method

– #1 Technique – Always delving deeper into my inner awareness training.

– Precisely speaking the words for the forms loud enough to hear.

– Listening.

– Writing, re-writing notes. Drawing and videoing oneself can also be used with the written notes.

– Reading the notes and other information.

– Physically doing the movements and forms.

– Developing new language skills.

– Visualizing movements, forms, notes, and other information.

– Consistently making healthy decisions and taking positive actions. Also learning from successes and missteps, and cleaning up missteps.

– Being enthusiastic, having fun, and enjoying the moment while working diligently.

February 1994

It's been five months since I started Phase I of my brain healing journey, and this is a great time to take stock. (The last 3 chapters) **Step by step, I continue delving deeper into my #1 technique – my inner awareness training. It's all about developing new ways to deepen my inner awareness – being aware of new and previously discovered areas; connections or reconnections in my body. I'm astonished how easy and fun my inner awareness and brain healing training is to do. For the first time since the TBI I'm working smarter, not harder.** I'm now aware and have made connections to more muscles, joints, etc., mostly in my legs, but also in my feet, arms, shoulders, chest, and back. As a result of my new level of inner awareness and connections, I'm remembering and owning more martial art forms, including new forms, other information, and my words are flowing a little bit better. My energy level has also increased; I'm having more good days, and I'm doing my brain healing training, and practicing with my workout buddies at school for longer periods of time. Physically, I'm a little bit stronger and flexible, but only very slightly more coordinated on the outside. In addition, step by step, I've had to purposefully readjust to my newly enhanced abilities: mentally, verbally, and physically, and of course, inner awareness. I love that readjusting to new levels and abilities is a regular part of my journey.

I've also experienced a tiny shift forward in the time delay between brain damage time and the foreign outside world time. I've gained a half-step towards being in the present time of the foreign outside world, and I've had to readjust my internal clock. Though inside I'm a bit more centered, I don't feel a connection with either world. What's interesting is I'm so used to the time delay world of brain damage that being in-between both worlds doesn't seem like much of an improvement. However, I'll take the forward progress. I also understand time, but still prefer to tell time by the seasons and the weather; it's more natural. It's easy to sense the temperature has warmed up a bit, and see that daylight is lasting a little longer. I've also noticed the bald eagles are beginning to get restless; next month, in March, they'll fly north.

Another great benefit of my inner awareness training is this wonderful, positive feeling of *fullness* in my brain when I finish my brain healing training for the day. This fullness is a welcome change and vastly different than the yucky feeling of always being dead in the head or overwhelmed in my brain. The *brain fullness* lets me know I've made good progress, and it's time to chill and maybe get something to eat. I've learned from my missteps that if I continue to push, it will set me back and hinder my progress. Again, trying to find a balance of how much brain healing training to do, practicing with my workout buddies at school, taking martial art classes, volunteering, and the responsibilities of daily activities is quite a challenge. Once again, my gut is letting me know, to improve my inner awareness; I need to continue doing *all* these activities.

In addition, I don't need as much sleep, yet my energy level continues to improve. Unfortunately, many mornings I still wake up with the same nightmare, which started about nine months after the accident, that's when I began to remember dreams and nightmares. The nightmare is I'm imprisoned in my brain, and not able to think, remember, and speak right, and my life has been completely destroyed. I wake up and realize it's not a nightmare – this is my life. Crap. Dejection turns into excitement as I turn over and see my brain healing training pants and comfortable t-shirt I'll wear for the day.

How do I find balance with my brain healing training and everything else? Well, I absolutely know everything I'm doing is deepening my inner awareness and accelerating the pace of my brain healing journey. Although, I'm still not sure how much to do and how fast to move forward; this is an interesting quandary and a skill I need to own. I believe a person with an intact brain would have a difficult time finding balance. I wish there was a map or someone to guide me. But, there isn't a map or person to lead me and wishing will not help. Instead of focusing on what's not working, I consciously change my perspective. Finding balance in my journey is a positive challenge and *It's Easy* to find a solution.

With my mind-set squared away, it's easy to remember even more benefits. I'm really hungry after working out, eating healthier, and I'm finally aware when I'm hungry. I'm also not using the dark sunglasses and ear plugs as much. The thought of losing my rock star status puts a smile on my face; what a great trade off.

In addition, my notes for my forms are a little clearer and more precise. When I forget a move, or as my workout buddies at the school say, have a brain fart, most of the time I need to fix my notes. I've gotten into the habit of regularly updating all my notes; re-writing them in more detail and so they're easy to read. At first, I thought my writing had improved because of my brain healing training. Although this is true to a point, my writing has also improved because, as a martial artist, I see, do, and understand my old and new forms, and information better than when I started.

In five months, I've made outstanding progress. But, and it is a big but. There isn't a dent in the thick, blurry glass wall, and in my minds-eye, I continue climbing in complete darkness in the never-ending hole; hopefully, in the right direction. I don't understand why there isn't at least a little nick in the prison in my brain or some light in the never-ending hole? How come I'm a little bit better in all areas of my life, yet some evenings I'm really tired, and the challenges of TBI come roaring back? When I look in the mirror, why do I still see brain damage in my eyes and on my face? Why haven't I experienced any more brain awakenings? Why are my outer movements still awkward, yet inside my body, I aware of my muscles, joints, etc. trying to get in sync? How come when I do my brain healing training at home and my volunteer job as a horse leader, I have more confidence and trust my memory, and I'm usually right? But, I don't trust my memory when I train with my workout buddies at school, who all have intact brains, especially the students with CD-ROM brains; they have excellent memories. The lack of confidence with my memory is vastly different than anything I've ever experienced. **I thought for sure when my memory came back I would totally trust it.**

Rather than focus on the negatives, I change my mind-set. By continuing to delve deeper into my precious inner awareness training, I've made extraordinary progress. So many tasks are easier to do compare to before starting Phase I of my brain healing journey. Although there isn't any change in the thick, blurry glass wall, one of my measuring sticks. I have great hope and believe I'll continue improving by leaps and bounds as long as I *keep delving deeper into my precious inner awareness training.*

Before I continue blazing my brain healing trail, I look at why I'm making phenomenal progress. Of course, the answer is I'm delving deeper into my inner awareness and brain healing training and *simultaneously* applying *all* my techniques. Well, the brain works *simultaneously.* The brain doesn't do one thing at a time; it *simultaneously* does numerous tasks. The brain is like the conductor of an orchestra – doing multiple tasks, layered one on top of another, forming an organism that works in *perfect harmony*.

I wonder about the approach at rehab and why it didn't heal my brain. Though I have the highest regard for the people at rehab, there is a separation in their approach. Physical therapy works the body while speech therapy works on the mental skills: verbal, writing, memory, reading, study skills, etc. Even occupational therapy, the most diverse therapy, has a separation in its approach. If all the outside rehabilitation techniques are applied simultaneously, they still will not work because their approach is an *outer focus for an inner problem*. It's crystal clear. Trying to push outside intellectual knowledge and techniques through the thick, blurry glass wall does not work and is not the solution to completely heal my brain. Information is not transformation. (Again, I use the analogy of an engine and computer to put this into context.) If an engine is clogged or running rough, or a computer is slow, I wouldn't add more fuel into the engine, or input more information or videos into a computer and expect the problem to be fixed. It's the same with the brain. Inputting more outside, intellectual information and techniques into a busted brain and expecting it to break through the thick, blurry glass wall is nuts. *The solution must come from inside.*

The only pathway that's working is my inner awareness and brain healing training; it is a positive, self perpetuating cycle and has become such a natural part of me that it's play. In my gut, I get a strong sense. Don't focus on how the outer movements look, the outer benefits, or the outer success. I need to keep discovering other ways to delve deeper into my precious inner awareness method – how my inner body moves, works, and connects.

12

FACING
OBSTACLES
INSIDE AND OUT

The vast majority of my martial art training is with the external martial arts, also known as the hard styles. The power for external martial art movements come from the muscles and the moves are usually powerful, fast, and large. However, the external martial arts are only one-half of martial arts. The internal martial arts are known as the soft styles, and the power for the movements comes from *chi,* not from the muscles. Supposedly, chi is the essential energy that exists in all living things. But, I don't believe in chi or the internal martial arts; all of it sounds new age, and I'm definitely not a new age, crystal kind of person. I like things concrete, things I can experience, not the BS of new age magic. On the other hand, I know very little about the internal arts, meditation, and chi; there's so much to learn and the saying is ten years is a good beginning. Could the internal martial arts, meditation, and chi help me delve deeper into my inner awareness training, and are they powerful enough to break through the prison in my brain? I don't know. I decide to stay skeptical and be open.

Chi kung postures are usually slow, gentle movements or still postures. Tai chi or the grand ultimate fist are a series of connected movements that range from very slow to explosively fast and powerful, and from miniscule to very large. Basic meditation is done in static postures: sitting, standing, and other postures which cultivates and enhances the chi. But, the process of cultivating and enhancing chi is a very slow, step by step, process that takes patience, time, and must not be rushed. While doing the internal martial arts and meditating I need to place the tip of my tongue on the roof of my mouth just behind my front teeth with a little saliva to act as a bridge. Although I don't understand why the tip of my tongue needs to be in this position, I try it and it feels really weird and right at the same time. I trust that one day I will understand this very unusual requirement. In addition, it is crucial that people who are mentally unstable are not taught how to circulate chi because they could lose what little grasp of reality they have left. I don't totally understand why mentally unstable people are not taught this technique; again, I trust in time I will. Thankfully, I'm mentally stable; I just have a busted brain.

The sun is up and it's a beautiful Colorado morning. I begin my morning brain healing training by trying to meditate, but it's very confusing and my heart is just not into it. There is a lot to meditation: breathing patterns, how to breathe, where to breathe to, what to focus on, different acupuncture points, when is the best time to meditate, how long to wait to eat before and after meditating, cleansing breaths, when to swallow, how to hold your hands, what to wear, having good hygiene, preparing a meditation area, and using a timer.

Meditation is boring, it's too time consuming, there's too much to do, and it will take too long to get the results. I decide not to take the time to own mediation; it is too much work. Immediately, I have a gut sense that I need to break down mediation into a simple, step by step, process just like I've done with everything else in my brain healing journey. Simplifying meditation will make it easier to understand, and more importantly, it will help me delve deeper into my precious inner awareness training. But, I do not believe in mediation. Even though I'm extremely skeptical, I decide to be open and practice meditation, a little. With great reservation I also try a few common chi kung postures and a tai chi form. Though there's an abundance of chi kung postures to choose from, I select a few and practice them diligently with the method that's taught at the school. But, I'm not making *any* progress with meditation, the chi kung postures, or the tai chi form.

When I go to the school, I respectfully ask the instructors for an explanation about the internal martial arts, meditation, and chi. The answers are extremely complicated and vague. I politely ask the question in a different way; again, the answers are just as mysterious. At first, I think it's the TBI; however, when other students, all with intact brains, ask similar questions, they too get the same confounding explanations. Afterwards, I ask each student if they understood what the instructors said. They tell me no. Then, they almost reiterate the confusing explanations given by the instructors. Next, I ask students from lower belt levels to upper Black Belt levels if they regularly practice, or in the future will they practice the internal martial arts and meditation. The vast majority of students say no; the internal martial arts, meditation, and chi are too hard to understand, and it will take too long to even begin to grasp the basics. A few upper Black Belts say they'll practice, but they don't believe they'll make much progress.

Could the internal martial arts, meditation, and chi be that baffling and difficult to master or is it the teaching at this school? For the first time I examine the instruction at this martial art school. First, it's easy to see that their main focus is the external martial arts; although, they do teach the internal martial arts and meditation. Second, they teach forms, a few applications, and some history of each form. Then, it's up to each student to investigate the movements and forms in order to understand the martial essence. However, they do not teach how to investigate and decipher the essence of the forms. Third, they teach in a very complicated and confusing manner. Once again, I think it's the TBI, until I talk with my workout partners and higher-ranking Brown and Black Belts, including students with CD-ROM brains. Their experience is the same as mine.

What is most interesting is when the instructors are out of town, and the assistants teach the classes, there is a massive improvement in the level of teaching and comprehension across all the classes. The assistants teach the forms and other information simply and exceptionally well; everything is very easy to understand. I make a decision that when I teach my method to heal the brain, I will teach everything simply and so it is easy to understand, especially my precious inner awareness training.

Should I go to another martial art school? I consider my previous martial art experience and my search of schools in the area. *Changing schools or adjusting my focus to understand the martial essence of forms will not help me discover a solution to the TBI. Martial art schools are going to teach martial arts. Once again, there isn't a school of any kind, organization, or person in the world who can help me discover a solution to TBI. My gut is letting me know to stick with my course of action – the solution is inside me; keep delving deeper into my precious inner awareness training.*

I decide to continue being respectful and learn the techniques of martial arts, acupuncture, and other tools. Then, I'll transform these tools into positive, healthy new techniques for my brain healing journey; basically I'll utilize them to delve deeper into my inner awareness training. There's another reason to stay at the school, I love the enthusiasm, camaraderie, and positive attitude of my workout partners; they inspire me.

With that squared away, I'm back to my original dilemma. Plain and simple: what are the internal martial arts, meditation, and chi, how do they work, and precisely how do I do them? I continue my search, reading internal martial art books and magazines. Regrettably, they're also written in this mysterious vagueness and complexity; even the CD-ROM students have a difficult time understanding them.

People suggest I watch martial art movies that depict the powerful chi energy. But all I find is mystery and hype of chi's *other worldly power*. At the end of the movie there's always a big fight scene. The master barely touches the bad guy with his super powerful internal strike, and instantly, the villain flies across the room while this very weird music is played. The music is supposed to further dramatize the master's explosive chi. The scoundrel smashes into the wall and is enveloped in a cloud of dust. As the dust is clearing, bricks fall on top of his head. Their portrayal of chi is absolutely ludicrous; I can see the wire that yanks the bad guy back as he's struck.

To make matters worse, there are real world prejudices and secrecy about the internal martial arts, meditation, and chi. Over and over again, many martial art instructors and students say, write, and teach that Chinese people will cultivate and enhance their chi first, and that they will *always* be better than anyone else at the internal martial arts. It will also take at least ten years before a person will begin to experience chi, and only a few lucky Chinese people will ever be taught the "correct way with all the secrets." I smell fear – plain ole small-minded bigotry. People can try to dress up their words, but they still reek of fear, and I disregard all of it as BS. Again, *every time* a person puts themselves or another person down (including politicians, celebrities, organizations, etc., and even objects), they are loudly announcing to the world how fear-filled they are, and precisely what they think and feel about themselves, not anyone or anything else. People can disagree, agreeable, and respectfully.

I've hit wall after wall trying to learn and practice the internal martial arts, meditation, and chi, and I still don't know if they're powerful enough to break through the prison in my brain. Plain and simple, what are the internal martial arts, meditation, and chi, how do they work, and precisely how do I do them?

I change my mind-set by asking a different question. How badly do I want to completely liberate myself from the prison in my brain and be reconnected? How much do I want to own the internal martial arts, meditation, chi, and any other technique that will help me in my brain healing journey to delve deeper into my inner awareness training? I'm either persevering forwards or backwards; there is no such thing as staying the same. So, what's it going to be?

I decide to apply the powerful technique of *It's Easy*, and immediately, an enormous determination rises within me. To hell with people's prejudices, doubts, and even my own bloody doubts about the internal martial arts, meditation, chi, or any other BS that gets in my way. I will not allow anyone or anything to confine, define, or control me. *It's Easy* to learn, be aware, and experience the tools and methods of the internal martial arts, meditation, and chi. Then, I'll simplify and transform them into techniques that are easy to understand and apply to my brain healing training, which will help me to, *step by step, delve deeper into my precious my inner awareness training. It's Easy.*

13

LIKE A DUCKLING TAKING TO WATER EARLY SPRING 1994

Boldly, I state my intentions. *It's Easy* to own the internal martial arts, meditation, and chi! *It's Easy* to do my best and figure out my next right step in delving deeper into my inner awareness training! *It's Easy* to develop a positive, healthy method that will completely heal and enhance my brain, better than before the TBI! *It's Easy, and it's going to get easier!*

I select a few common chi kung postures and a tai chi form. Rather than practice with the method taught at the martial art school or in books. I choose the only path that's working, and working phenomenally well – my inner awareness training. *First,* I become and stay aware of my inner body – how my muscles, joints, etc. are moving and connecting while doing the movements. Immediately, my inner awareness massively improves; I'm aware of my inner body in a *whole new level* than when I do my external martial art forms. I'm aware of my muscles, joints, etc. moving, connecting, and working in unison, but something is missing. I deepen my inner awareness by intensifying my focus to a small area in my right upper arm. Little by little, it becomes natural to be aware of the muscles working more in unison; again, it's different than doing the external martial art movements. *I am astounded at how comfortable it is to be aware of my inner body while doing the internal martial art movements; it feels like I'm making my way home.*

Next, I focus to an adjacent area in my arm and how muscles etc. are connecting and moving. I'm pleasantly surprised how easier and faster it is to be aware; it's like I'm getting in sync with my inner body *in* a whole new level. I barely start to be aware of another area in my arm, and almost immediately, I'm aware of the muscles and joints connecting and flowing. Deep in my gut, I get a sense that my inner body, and brain has been waiting for me to delve deeper into my inner awareness training in order to make these reconnections. I love, love, love my inner awareness training.

Day after day, and week after week, I persistently delve deeper into my precious inner awareness training by practicing my chi kung postures, tai chi, very little meditation, and my external martial art forms. My results are stunning. My inner body is beginning to work in harmony. I'm also not using the ear plugs and wrist brace while doing my chi kung postures, tai chi, meditation, some conditioning and stretching, and most daily activities. My wrist has a little more range of motion. Also, I've permanently put away my dark sunglasses, except when I'm outside on sunny days.

A few weeks pass, and I'm getting concerned I've hit the wall of TBI again. I'm having difficulty remembering the longer sequence of movements of a tai chi form. This doesn't make sense because the tai chi form is done so much slower than the more dynamic and faster external forms which are easier for me to own. I'm a low level Brown Belt; I should be able to own the slower movements of tai chi. I continue practicing, but no matter how much I apply my inner awareness training and brain healing techniques, including my Simultaneous Brain Learning Method, I'm not able to own the tai chi form.

I talk with my workout buddies and senior students at school. They all laugh; some let out a huge belly laugh. One person sums up what all the others have said. "Cathy, everyone – including people with CD-ROM brains has a difficult time remembering internal martial art forms. This is just the way it is." At first the explanation seems backwards, but the more I practice the internal martial arts, the more I know it's true. When it comes to internal martial arts, how I think it should be is usually the exact opposite of how it works.

I try to meditate, but it's still boring. Meditation doesn't have the coolness of my chi kung postures and tai chi, and it certainly doesn't have the pop and pizzazz of my external martial art forms. Again, I have a gut sense that meditation will help me in my journey. I decide to keep meditating though it will still be a lesser pursuit.

Next, I get a huge gut sense to slow down each movement in my chi kung postures and tai chi form. *I need to become aware of how my lower inner body: inner feet, then legs, hips, and waist, moves my upper inner body: inner trunk, then arms, hands, and head.* I start as always – aware of my inner body. Move by move, I'm surprised at how easy it is to be aware of the flow, movement, and connections of the inner movements in my feet, legs, hips, then waist; it feels like a foundation is being built within me. In some ways, this foundation reminds me of rooting, but it's much more than rooting. In addition, my outer focus, energy level, clarity, memory etc. has naturally deepened and improved a bit. I also sense that I'm trying to tap into a natural, powerful, calm, centered energy within me. Describing this energy is challenging, which makes sense, because like my inner awareness training; this energy must be experienced; it's not an intellectual exercise.

Intrigued and very encouraged, I continue practicing and become aware of an ever so slight flow of energy moving through me. *I have never felt this good working out.* I finish my morning brain healing training, and for the first time, I'm able to do my inner awareness training in *all* my daily activities without having to consciously be aware of my inner body. In addition, my inner awareness, outer focus, energy level, clarity, memory etc. continues to deepen and improve. Yeaha, another giant leap forward in my brain healing journey and life!

My next right step in my inner awareness training is literally stepping using the *9 points of the foot.* My first *inner* connection is the center of my heel; then, I slowly roll my bare foot to the outside heel, top outside edge, ball of the foot, and grasp the ground with my five toes. In the beginning, being aware of my inner body while stepping, rolling, and grasping the earth with my bare feet feels strange. However, just like every other technique, with time and effort, it gets easier; then, it becomes natural to be inwardly aware. Again, my benefits are outstanding; I am more in the present from the, inside and out, and I'm a little more balanced, rooted, and coordinated. Once again, I sense my body and brain have been waiting for me to deepen my inner awareness by simultaneously utilizing all of my brain healing techniques.

I get a brilliant idea to do my chi kung postures, tai chi, and meditation using earplugs. My hope is the earplugs will further enhance my inner awareness, but this is a humongous mistake. Instead of being an asset, the ear plugs are blocking me from deepening my inner awareness. In addition, listening to music using headphones does not help. I permanently let go of my ear plugs; I've learned everything I can from them a long time ago.

A few mornings later while doing a chi kung posture, I experience a gentle tingling energy *in* my fingertips then it stops. Although this is really cool, I don't know what just happened. I end my morning brain healing training, and I am beyond thankful that, on my own, I remembered and did my chi kung postures and tai chi form.

I look out the window; spring is in full swing, everything is green. The magpies with their beautiful black and white bodies and iridescent long tail feathers are in the trees and on the lawn looking for breakfast. I hear a woodpecker loudly tapping on a tree in the backyard. Of course, the sparrows are having their usual lengthy morning squabble in the apple tree. A few seconds later the woodpecker, a stunning red shafted northern flicker, flies in front of the window; his salmon-colored feathers are gorgeous. He lands in a large tree in the front yard, and again, loudly taps on the tree. WOW, I was just doing my brain healing training and it was *easy* to be aware and keep my focus on my training. I wasn't distracted by any outside noise, and I wasn't sidetracked by the noise from the electronic devices in the room which are off. This is monumental; my inner and outer focus has improved big time; I love my inner awareness training!

Walking down the spiral stairs, I inwardly celebrate this historical achievement when my stomach lets me know I'm getting hungry. But, I need to wait 45 minutes before I can eat, go to the bathroom, or sit down. Otherwise the chi I cultivated from my internal training will be lost. Even though I still don't believe in chi, I'm open. While waiting to eat I plan my day; including, more brain healing training, taking Maja on a longer and more challenging hike on the south side of Mt. Sanitas in the afternoon, and other activities. Next, I make some phone calls; then, I make an excellent breakfast, my favorite meal of the day. I absolutely love, love, love breakfast! In the afternoon, in the middle of a wonderful hike, I realize all my celebrations for my brain healing journey have occurred mostly inside. Is this a clue? I don't know.

Weeks later, I have even more interesting experience with this energy inside my body. While doing a common chi kung posture, I again experience a wonderful, gentle tingling *in* my fingertips and my inner hands feel warmer. In addition, not only am I aware of this energy, I'm aware of deeper and more inner connections with muscles, joints, etc. This is so beyond cool! I believe I know what's happening with the tingling *in* my fingertips, but it couldn't be happening this soon and be this easy to do. I open my eyes, shake my hands, and return to my chi kung posture. Once again, the energy pulsates *inside* my fingertips. Is someone playing a trick on me? I open my eyes, but I'm in my home alone with my dog who's sound asleep. I close my eyes, take a deep, slow breath, and resume my posture. *The sensation of tingling and warmth returns.* **I smile; this is my first confirmation of chi!** *Could experiencing chi be as simple and easy as delving deeper into my inner awareness training? I believe so! I let success go to my head, and instantly, my wonderful sensation of chi disappears. In my mind, I hear a mentor, "Stomp on your ego with both feet." I switch my mind-set; be humble and stay open.*

Immediately, I become aware of my inner body and the sensations of chi returns. Being aware of chi in my inner fingers and hands is completely natural; I feel like a duckling taking to water. Chi feels like a soft ball of energy, or a less dense version of silly putty, it also feels like two big magnets between my hands. I start playing with my chi trying to figure out how far I can pull my hands apart before losing the sensation of chi. My hands are almost the width of my shoulders when the sensation of chi dissipates. Slowly, I bring my hands together; they feel like they're being drawn together by a big magnet. When my hands are about five inches apart the chi prevents them from getting closer. I'd have to use my muscles to generate force to get them closer. But, that would defeat the purpose of my inner awareness and the internal martial arts training.

Playing with chi is impressive and beautiful; my chi is literally moving *in* my hands, especially *in* my fingertips. The more I play with my chi, the further I'm able to delve deeper into my precious inner awareness training, which has increased my inner, then outer focus, energy, clarity, memory, etc. to whole new levels.

A week later, I have another wonderful experience with my chi while practicing another common chi kung posture. As I shift my stance from my right side to left; my left inner body is full of chi while my right side feels lighter, not in weight, but in energy. I shift my stance to the right and the chi transfers to the right; it feels like I'm shifting from one time zone to another.

In a very short amount of time, my inner awareness has naturally deepened to many new levels. I've also gone from being a complete skeptic about chi, to becoming aware and experiencing chi. I continue practicing and it feels like I'm plugging into many, many areas of energy inside my body, which has raised me to another whole new, deeper level of inner awareness, clarity, energy, memory, etc. In addition, the gap between my inner world and the foreign outside world continues to close, step by step. Now, it is second nature to readjust my internal clock.

I share my experiences of chi and the internal martial arts with my workout buddies at school and other students, but I sense and see their doubts. I tell them not to be swayed by what happened to me or anyone else. Stay skeptical, keep an open mind, and give the internal martial arts your absolute best effort; then, you'll know if chi and the internal martial arts are real or not. They tell me they're focusing on their external martial forms and testing to their next belt level. I accept their decisions and continue to focus on my training and healing.

At this time, I had no idea that being aware of chi would profoundly surge my brain healing journey forward, step by step. I will discover so much more about chi, which will help me to delve deeper into my precious inner awareness training, and it will open doors to make even more connections in my inner body. However, now it's time to take stock of some of my remarkable improvements and some very interesting luxury challenges.

LIFE IS ALWAYS A BALANCING ACT
EARLY SUMMER
1994

This is a great time to take stock of my brain healing journey. It's only been a little over nine months since I've started Phase I and my progress is beyond exceptional. My inner awareness training is off the charts phenomenal, and the powerful, peaceful, dynamic energy of chi is invigorating. I own more forms, and my verbal and physical skills continue to improve. It is so much easier to speak each movement out loud while I'm doing forms at home, with my workout buddies at school, and in class. I am thoroughly enjoying a huge increase in energy, I'm having more fun, and I'm doing even more: brain healing training, martial art classes, training with my workout buddies at school, and activities at home and socially. Even my dog is benefiting from all my phenomenal improvements; we're taking longer, more challenging hikes and exploring new hiking areas. With all my outstanding progress, I now have more opportunities.

Recently I've been asked to help out at the martial art school. I've been given the key to open and close the school when the instructors are out of town or running late. I run the desk by my self; this is unheard of for a Brown Belt to be given such a great responsibility. I sign up new students, handle all financial transactions (cash, check, credit card, and receipts), balance the daily receipts, prepare the deposit, and answer the phone and questions from students and perspective students. These are just a few of my responsibilities. In addition, while the instructors and some students travel throughout China, I am in charge of running the school for two weeks. On top of all my other responsibilities, I need to make sure all the assistants teach the classes well and everything runs smoothly. With the mind-set of *It's Easy* and my precious inner awareness training, I do an excellent job with everything. Each time I finish all my responsibilities at the school, I am really tired, sleep well, and the next day, I do my brain healing training and everything else with ease. I've come a long way from not knowing what numbers meant and how to count; to easily handling financial transactions. From not being able to speak a simple two to three word sentence, to easily and quickly speaking on the phone and handling questions from a multitude of people speaking, at the same time.

I love that I am improving by huge leaps and bounds, and now, I have luxury challenges, which are pretty good things to handle considering where I came from. My first, luxury challenge, which I continue to deal with, is I'm constantly trying to balance my brain healing training, learning new forms, testing to my next belt level, training with my workout buddies at school (all of them have intact brains), volunteering, and all my other activities. Although I don't want to test at the supersonic speed like most students, I don't want to slow down and lose interest in my training. Another part of the challenge is pushing my self to keep up physically and mentally with my workout buddies at school, which has been enormously helpful. It is refreshing to be around people who are working on improving themselves, who focus on finding solutions, and who set the bar high on attaining excellence. On the other hand, because of my bad habit of being impatient and pushing myself, I have to deal with some down time in my brain healing training. This amount of time varies depending on how much I worked out and less on the TBI.

Trying to balance everything is a massive job; heck, this would be a huge challenge for people with intact brains.

The second, luxury challenge which continues to plague me is a lack of confidence with my memory when I work out with students with intact brains at school. It's crystal clear I trust my memory when I train by myself at home and at the school, and volunteering at the riding center. But, when I practice forms with my workout buddies at school, especially the ones with CD-ROM brains, **I ask memory questions even when I know the correct answers. When I hear the answer that I already knew, I say out loud, "I knew that! WHY do I keep asking questions I know the answers to?"** When I'm tired, I ask even more questions and get more frustrated after hearing the answer that I already knew. Then again, every student asks memory questions, especially about those pesky transitional moves. What's interesting, in a weird way, is that after I've asked a memory question and gotten the answer, invariably someone with an intact brain quietly thanks me for asking the question they wanted to ask but were afraid to. It sort of feels good that a person with an intact brain was having a brain fart and I already knew the answer. But, the lack of confidence with my memory when around people with intact brains is absolutely frustrating. **I was 100% certain once my memory improved, I'd be able to trust it – just as I had pre-TBI.** Could I be like Pavlov's dog? I don't know. I also don't know how to trust my memory, especially when I know I'm right. Hopefully, the solution is also inside me.

Despite all my remarkable progress, the thick, blurry glass wall is still completely intact. Rather than focus on why there isn't at least a dent in the prison in my brain, *I decide to accept that it no longer matters.* Focusing on the "why's and the how come's" is a waste of time and energy which will only take me off-course. My number one job is to keep delving deeper into my inner awareness training in order to completely liberate and reconnect myself. Period.

I also put my luxury challenges into perspective. Are you

kidding? This is Friggin Awesome! At least now, I have memory and usually I'm right. In some ways, I think it's good that I'm not totally self-assured regarding my memory. Hopefully, I'll stay humble and hungry. As for balancing the tremendous drive to completely free myself from the prison in my brain and be reconnected; I don't know if pushing my self is a good thing, a bad thing, or both, but it's a heck of a lot better than drooling. What I'm doing is working extraordinarily well, and if it isn't broke, don't fix it.

With my mind-set squared away, it's time to figure out my next right step. Are the internal martial arts and chi powerful enough to break through the thick, blurry glass wall, and will I be able to generate enough chi? In my gut, I know it's going to take a tremendous amount of power to unlock the prison in my brain. The only thing that's felt powerful enough is the movements from the external martial art forms. Do I put my focus and precious energy into the internal martial arts where ten years is a good beginning? Or, do I channel my focus into the external martial arts where I'm getting great results right now?

Well, my main goal is to always delve deeper into my inner awareness training and the internal and external martial arts have done an outstanding job. However, the external arts are strengthening my body while challenging my mind. On the other hand, the internal martial arts and chi feels like home. But, I've just scratched the surface of the internal martial arts, and I have some major concerns. I don't think the movements are powerful enough to break through the prison in my brain. The moves seem too fluffy, compared to the strength I experience and see with the external strikes. Though I'm at a crossroads, it's an easy decision. There's no way I'm going to wait ten years to make a good beginning with the internal martial arts. I am going to focus on the tangibles of the external martial arts. However, I will keep an open mind about the internal martial arts and continue practicing them, though not as much.

My last decision puts a huge smile on my face; I will test to 1st Degree Black next spring 1995, about nine months away.

Immediately, I have a huge gut sense that the external martial arts and attaining my 1st Degree Black Belt is *not* the answer to TBI. Although I don't know it, very soon I will plateau in my inner awareness training using any external movements. There is only so much inner awareness one can experience from the muscles, joints, etc. while doing any external movements. Even though my decisions don't set well with me, I decide to move forward in my external approach and testing to 1st Degree Black Belt because I don't believe there are any other viable solutions – this is the trail I will blaze.

14

AN
EXTRAORDINARY
TURN OF EVENTS

On my own I'm having a great time practicing my Brown Belt forms at the school, when I notice a fellow student watching me. He's a gentle, quiet man, with an intact brain who's easily able to remember forms and other information. I finish a form, and he sincerely asks. "I'm having trouble remembering some moves, especially the transitional moves from a different form than you're working on. Will you help me?" He tells me the form and some of his sticking areas.

I'm shocked – there's no way he's asking me, a no-brainer, memory questions. I turn to my right to see who he's talking to; no one's there. As I turn to my left, I quickly glance at him to see if he's messing with me. Again, I sense his sincerity. I finish my panoramic view; no one is behind me. I smile at him and joke to myself – who's the one with a TBI?

The doubts – fears start rearing their ugly heads. Instead of focusing on the fact that I know the form, and I've made phenomenal progress, I feed the doubts. I'm a Brown Belt who's got a TBI. What happens if I get flustered? I won't be able to say the words right or do the movements correctly. Arrgh, the scourge of TBI; this friggin lack of confidence with memory is breathing down my neck. Rather than stepping up and helping the man based on the truth of my abilities, I make a decision based on the lies of the doubts. I point to another student and say, "Hey man, see that guy over there, he'd be better at showing you the form." I let out a huge sigh of relief as I watch him walk over and ask the man for help. On my own, I continue practicing my forms. A few minutes later the man returns with the same question; he needs help with a form. I ask him why the guy didn't help. He just shrugs. I make a decision to help him and say, "Okay man, I'll help you with the form." *I take a few seconds* to visualize the form, paying close attention to his sticking areas, and my notes, including some Chinese words and phrases. Next, I say to myself, *It's Easy* to teach this form and I will do the best job I can.

We bow and begin the first of three sections of the form. I'm doing what I normally do; enthusiastically, I'm speaking each movement out loud while doing the form. When we come to his first sticking point, I purposefully slow down my physical pace and place special emphasis on my words. I glance over to make sure he's keeping up. Instead of paying attention, he's giving me this weird look. Without missing a beat I say, "Hey man, focus on what you're doing." *I chuckle to myself; I've just told a person with an intact brain to focus! This is amazing – who would have thought I'd be telling a person with an intact brain to focus! While mentally patting myself on the back, I almost lose my place in the form, and remind myself to focus.*

We finish the first section of the form and I'm feeling really good. I'm excited as I explain how speaking the movements out loud while doing the form helps me to remember and do the form better. Exuding from him is disbelief. I smile and say, "It's okay if you have doubts. The only way I believed speaking the movements out loud worked was by experiencing it." My explanation seems to ease some of his doubts. I ask if he has any questions; he tells me no. Next I ask, "While we're going through the first section again, how about if you speak each movement loud enough for you to hear." It's easy to sense his hesitancy. To ease his nervousness I share, "I was embarrassed the first time I spoke the movements out loud and I was by myself." We laugh. I say, "Laughing is good, it takes away some of that uneasy energy. So what do you think about trying to speak each movement out loud? What have you got to lose?" He thinks it over and nods in agreement.

We start the first section again, and I hear him having trouble choosing the words for each movement. While we're doing the form, I quickly tell him, "You can repeat my words." As soon as I finish my sentence, I completely lose my place in the form. Immediately, I realize a couple of things. First, I need to focus on what I'm doing, especially with something as complex as teaching, while doing the form, speaking each movement out loud, and most importantly, my inner awareness training. Second, I'm not able to keep my outer focus on another person while doing all these tasks. Not yet.

Again, we start the first section, and when we finish, he is overjoyed as he says. "It's almost effortless to remember the moves by speaking the words out loud! I'm shocked how simple and easier it is, but I don't have all the right words for each movement, how do you say all the words while doing the form?" "Practice, practice, practice. Let's get down to basics. First, it's okay to repeat my words. Later, you can come up with your own words for each movement or you can use mine. Whatever works; no stress man." He agrees. I ask if he has any other questions; he doesn't.

Next I ask, "Do you want to learn other techniques that have helped me to remember and accomplish so much more?" His smile widens, "Yes." I give him a brief overview of my #1 brain healing technique, my inner awareness method, and some of my Simultaneous Brain Learning Method. Of course, I don't talk about my brain healing journey, and I don't call them my brain healing techniques.

I share how my inner awareness training specifically helps me and how cool and fun it is to do. "While simultaneously blocking, punching, and kicking, and doing every movement in all my forms, I'm aware of how my muscles, joints, etc. are moving and connecting. Being aware of my inner body helps me to own the movements, then the forms, and it is so simple and a blast. Even though my outer movements don't flow and my stances aren't as deep as other students, the more I practice being aware of my muscles, joints, etc., the more aware I become and the more I improve. It quickly became natural to be aware of my inner body which, step by step, made it a little easier to remember and do my forms."

He leans in, looking directly into my eyes. Now, he's looking to see if I'm messing with him. He says, "I don't know about all that; it seems a bit much." I smile and say, "Good you're skeptical, so was I. Stay skeptical, but keep an open mind. Remember, you had doubts about speaking the words out loud and look how well it worked. What have you got to lose by *simultaneously* adding more techniques? If you're willing to try, you've got to *always* do your best; half-ass attempts won't get the job done. Remember, Kung Fu means mastery through time and effort. A person can be Kung Fu as a martial artist, a watercolor painter, a chef, a computer technician, a mathematician, a salesperson etc. You can also be Kung Fu at speaking the words for each movement, being aware of your inner body, and in time, simultaneously adding more techniques to help you become even more aware of your inner body. You've got to do *all* the work and give it everything you've got to get *all* the results."

Tentatively, he simultaneously blocks and strikes. It's easy to be aware and see the frustration building up as he keeps his focus on his outer hands and arms. Calmly I say, "Keep it simple. The simple approach is usually the most successful and the easiest to apply with something new. What gets in the way is thinking that it should be more difficult and complex. When I complicate things, my brain goes into overdrive, and I miss the simple solution that's right in front of me, or more to the point – inside me. Don't focus on your outer hands and feet. Focus on what's happening with *a* muscle in your right upper arm as you simultaneously block and punch."

A minute or so passes and his face lights up; his doubts are turning into recognition. He shares, "I've never really paid attention to this inner body stuff before, it feels like I'm trying to plug into my insides." After another minute he says, "My muscles are lengthening and contracting, but I'm not sure if I'm saying it right." I share, "Your words will most likely be a little different than mine, and every person will probably have their own unique way of describing what's happening inside their being; it's all good."

He continues to practice and admits, "I thought it'd be harder, and it would take much longer to be aware of my muscles, joints, etc., but it's easier than I thought." When he's naturally aware of his inner body while simultaneously blocking, punching, and kicking, I ask, "Are you ready to take the next step: be aware of your inner body: muscles, joints, etc. while doing the form and speaking the words out loud – *one move at a time?*" A huge smile comes over his face, and we begin the first of three sections of the form. Move by move, he easily completes the first section. We begin the second section, and I hear a group of four bullies loudly belittling other students on the other side of the room. *Exuding from the bullies is their negative energy gunk announcing how they think and feel about themselves, not anyone else.* The bullies continue mocking other students; then, the ring-leader raises his voice making sure everyone in the school can hear him; including the instructor, "We are the best martial artists in the school. None of you is half as good as us." Of course, the bullies aren't practicing forms like everyone else; they're just slacking and boasting. Bullies always want the easy way out. They're also looking for easy marks; they only go after people who let them. I don't understand why bullies and negativity are allowed in the school.

While we're working on the second section of the form, I see the bullies zoning in on us; with each step the smell of their fear intensifies. They walk in back of us, and the ring-leader again raises his voice so everyone in the school can hear. "Shut up! Just do the form!" He elbows his friend. "Why would anybody want to learn from *her* anyway?" The bullies let out a huge laugh. Calmly, I turn while standing up from my bow stance, and look each bully squarely in the eye. Although my heart is pounding and I'm feeling fear, I don't feed the fear. *I stay aware and connected to my inner being which calms and centers me.* My mind-set is no nonsense; I'm here to work, not to play friggin games. Inside, I know by staying calm and being non-threatening they're not going to do anything. Again, bullies are looking for easy targets; people who are afraid of them. Also, their "tells:" their fearful energy, sagging postures, and expressions on their faces give them away. They're not men; they're little kids with small minds existing in adult bodies. They're also not used to someone standing up and seeing them for who they are. This experience reminds me of working with horses and other animals. If I focus on and feed the fear, they'll try to take advantage. But, if I am aware, and stay aware and connected to my inner body, I'm calmer and more confident.

The bullies glance sideways at each other. A few seconds later, one of them looks up with a glint in his eye and says, "We didn't mean it. We were just kidding." Another jumps on the bandwagon, "Yea, yea we were just fooling around." They laugh, but it's the laugh of; did we get away with it?' I shake my head no. I think – Men take responsibility for themselves, they don't bully, and they don't put themselves, other people, or organizations, etc. down.

I return to training, and the quiet, gentle man, who had taken a few steps away from the bullies as I was standing up, very tentatively joins me while the scared bullies slink off to the corner of the room. Thankfully, with each step, the smell of their fear dissipates. A few minutes later, rather than practice their forms, I hear them trying to bully other students. In my mind, I make a plan to talk with each person individually in that bully group. My hope is by having respectful, positive conversations, and offering each person an opportunity to workout with positive, healthy people; they'll choose to take responsibility for their energy, words, and actions.

We finish the second section, and I sense the quiet, gentle man is having a hard time with what just happened. I ask, "Are you okay?" He shares, "I don't think I could have done what you did." Without hesitation I say, "I disagree." He's taken aback and asks, "What do you mean?" I share, "When you're aware of your inner body while also being aware of your surroundings, and a few other things, it's simple and so much easier to deal with people and situations. While the bullies were walking towards us, I was aware of them, and I also took into account their past energy, words, and actions. They're consistently negative – fearful. In this instance, I knew by handling the situation the way I did, they'd stop. In another circumstance, I might have handled it totally different. Each situation is unique.

Most people think bullies are angry, but when you break down anger, it's just plain ole fear. They are boys, not men, and they are full of fear. It might seem like bullies are putting down or ridiculing others. But, plain and simple, bullies and anyone who puts down a person or anything are announcing to the world how poorly they think and feel about themselves not anyone else. Fear rules their thinking, words, and actions. Every time a person gets angry, they're afraid. Now, don't get me wrong, fear is a natural human emotion. But, just because you feel fear doesn't mean you're in fear; it's what we do with fear that makes a world of difference."

I summarize how to: transform thinking, words, and actions, how it takes consistent practice to be positive or negative, and how to be responsible and constructive. Also, that's it is enormously easier and more enjoyable to be positive and persevere forward than backwards. Next, I share, "Attitude and focus are always a choice, a habit, and all habits can be changed. People who respect themselves, respect others. Even if a person disagrees with someone or something, they can disagree, agreeably and respectfully."

My new workout buddy takes a deep breath and quietly shares, "When I was in middle school, there were bullies who made people's lives a living hell, including mine. I didn't know how to deal with them, so I tried to stay out of their way, but that didn't always work. You've given me a lot of good things to think about and apply, and I appreciate everything you've shared." I smile and say, "Thanks. I'm beginning to cool down, how about we get back to the form?"

About half-way through the third and final section of the form, I quickly glance over to see how he's doing. He's smiling from ear to ear; there's a new vigor and poise as he speaks the words for the movements out loud while easily moving through his previous sticking points which puts an even bigger smile on my face.

We finish the form and his eyes are sparkling, and there's excitement in his voice, "I'm able to remember and do the movements so much better! It's easier and pretty amazing to be aware of my inner body, my muscles, joints, etc. and how they're moving and connecting!" I tell him, "Man, I'm proud of you, and I encourage you to keep delving deeper into being aware of your inner body and applying all the techniques simultaneously. Before you know it, you'll own them quicker than you can imagine which will help you with your forms and everything else. Trust me; if I can do it, *anybody can!*" He smiles and says, "I've learned more from you than just about anybody else." I reply, "You've helped me more, and in ways I'm not sure you can ever understand." I sense he's having a hard time believing me, but he's answered a question I've had for a bit. A person with an intact brain can quickly develop their inner awareness and improve as a whole. Before I return to practicing my forms on my own, I watch him flow through his entire form with ease.

What happens next is absolutely shocking. More and more students with intact brains are asking me memory questions about forms, other martial art information, and for help with their forms. Most times I help them; however, when I'm standing next to a workout buddy, especially ones with a CD-ROM brain, 95% of the time I defer to them, **even when I know the answers and I know the forms**.

I also offer to teach students how to develop inner awareness and my other brain healing techniques. Of course, I don't call them my brain healing techniques. Unfortunately, everyone politely declines; they want to learn forms and test to their next belt level. I accept their decisions.

I reflect on all the extraordinary turn of events. I love being able to do more, do it better, and in less time. It is absolutely phenomenally off the charts wonderful to help people, rather than being the one who always needs help. My inner awareness training continues to deepen my inner; then, outer focus, improve my memory, clarity, energy, verbal and physical skills, etc. I am also thoroughly enjoying owning more forms, and having a tiny bit more confidence with my memory when I'm around people with intact brains.

All of my positive, healthy experiences at the riding center, my past experiences at rehab, and unfortunately, many negative experiences at the martial art school have inspired me to make several decisions. First, if I'm ever in charge, in any situation, I will consciously create a positive and healthy environment where people are responsible and respectful with themselves and others. I know I did this after I got sober, but I've lost a step or two since the TBI. Second, in the future, I will choose wisely whom I teach; there's no room for inflated egos, negative attitudes, self-destructive behavior, and people not willing to do all the work, etc.

Also, I don't understand why the basic techniques, forms, and other information are taught so complicated at the martial art school, and why crucial martial art information is held back. Whatever the reason, it doesn't make any sense. Sharing all the experience and knowledge, and teaching it simply will strengthen the students, the teachers, the school, and the art. From this point forward, I will simply and clearly share everything I've learned and experienced in my brain healing journey, in martial arts, and in my life with people who are responsible for themselves and their energy, who have a positive mind-set, and who do *all* the work to get *all* the results. My hope is they will fully pass on to others what they've experienced, and be a positive asset with themselves, with others, and with the world.

Rather than having to wait for an opportunity, one presents itself. A student asks to train with my workout buddies and myself at a local park. Of course we agree because he has a great attitude, works hard, and helps others. We finish training, and we're talking about our workout, how we can improve, and of course, what we're going to eat. The new guy shares how he can't do some moves as good as one of the guys, who is the best martial artist of us all, and he doesn't think he'll improve as quickly or as much as others.

I wait for him to inhale and calmly say, "Please, don't talk about a fellow student that way." At first he's stunned, but he continues putting himself down. Once again, I wait for him to inhale and gently say, "Please, don't talk badly about someone I care about." He politely says, "I was talking about myself." Gently I say, "Please, don't talk poorly about someone I care about." His head cocks to the side and his eyes squint. I can tell he's trying to figure out what the heck is happening. Then, his whole body opens, exuding from him are acceptance, love, and respect. A warm smile comes over his face as he nods his head in appreciation. This is the last time I will hear him putting himself down. Without missing a beat, the group continues the conversation, and we get excited as we talk about food!

MEDITATION

My main focus is the external martial arts and preparing for my test to 1st Degree Black Belt which will take place months from now. However, I am being pulled in another direction. I am still drawn to the internal martial arts and chi, and I have huge gut sense to continue delving deeper into meditation – all of this will help me in my inner awareness and brain healing training. Even though I still have zero interest in mediating, *I continue getting the same gut sense; the internal martial arts, chi, and meditation will help me. I need to pay attention to this recurring gut sense; I do not want to miss my next right step because of my bias.* Though my time is limited because of my upcoming test, I decide to return to the basics of meditation and break it down so it's simple to understand and do; in order to delve deeper into my precious inner awareness training.

Plain and simple, meditation is focused thinking. Focusing on a task, a word, a phrase, or worrying about a problem or situation is meditating. Being aware of the breath or heartbeat is also meditating. There are significant benefits to meditating: it improves focus, increases oxygen levels, relieves stress, and helps to center one self, to name a few. The idea of totally quieting the mind is absolutely bogus, especially in the beginning when the focus is on the breath or heartbeat. As for being completely still, that's not going to happen because inside the body there are all kinds of movements: heart, lungs, other organs, blood, air, and everything else. There are many breathing patterns, postures, words, or sounds that can be used; I think of them as training wheels on a bike. However, once the breathing patterns and postures have become second nature; it's time to naturally utilize them without having to think of them.

Before I start meditating, I revisit the universal 4 Levels of Breathing to the upper, middle, and lower sections of the lungs, and the complete breath. I place the tip of my tongue with a little bit of saliva on the roof of my mouth just behind my teeth; this now feels right. Though I still don't understand why my tongue needs to be in this position for meditation and internal martial art training; again, I trust one day I will.

I place my palms on my upper and middle chest, and focus on breathing *only* into the upper level of my lungs, but with each inhale both hands rise. I keep focusing on breathing only into my upper lung when my mind sets off in another direction. My mind is thinking of everything else except meditation and it's not pleasant. I'm either in the past or the future. It's like my mind has a mind of its own. I'm experiencing the "chattering monkeys" of meditation. Gently, I say, "Cathy, be aware – and stay aware of breathing only into the upper level of the lungs."

I try to relax, and for a few seconds, my mind is quieter and seems to be following my direction. I get distracted by the sound of some electronic device in the room which is turned off. I refocus. Moments later, I'm listening to what sounds like a herd of sparrows fighting in the apple tree outside the closed window. Again, my mind wants to focus on everything else, except meditation. I sigh. It must be getting close for the timer to go off. Although I know its best not to look at the timer because it's distracting, I look anyway. I'm floored; it's only been a minute and one-half! This is going to be a long five minutes. Meditation reminds me of trying to train rambunctious puppies. I laugh, I had no idea *this is how my mind operates all the time.* How come it's easier to be aware and focused when I'm doing my chi kung postures and other forms? I'm moving while doing those forms, and the 4 levels of breathing and meditation is stationary; they are a higher phase of inner awareness training. Now that I know the problem and I can work on finding, then applying the solution.

The only way I'm going to own meditation is to keep persevering, but how do I quiet my mind? I decide to simplify everything by breaking down all the things I need to do to prepare for mediation and the actual meditation. I go back to my reliable technique, my inner awareness training, and apply the secret to owning any technique: practice, practice, and more practice. There isn't a magic wand or pill for owning a technique or activity; it takes time and effort. I've learned that taking short cuts or doing things half-ass is just a waste of time and energy and something I'm not willing to do.

First, I square away my mind-set. *It's Easy to own meditation, and it will become second nature just like everything else, which will help me to delve deeper into my precious inner awareness training.* I begin by being aware of my inner body which always centers me. Next, I place my palms on my upper and middle chest, and become a little aware of the breath going into the upper lungs. Although both hands are expanding, I'm now aware of the movement of my ribs. Day after day, I practice deepening my inner awareness while working on breathing only into my upper lungs. Breath by breath, my inner awareness deepens while my upper lungs fill a little more than my middle lungs. Again, I deepen my inner awareness, and my mind is slightly quieter which deepens my inner awareness even more. My inner awareness training continues to be a positive, self-perpetuating cycle.

Slowly, the squabbling birds, chattering monkeys, and everything else quiets down inside. I intently deepen my inner awareness and become aware of other parts of my upper chest. There are connections between my ribs that are expanding and contracting. Breath by breath, my inner awareness deepens, and breathing into my upper lungs becomes fuller and deeper. I remove my hands and continue breathing only into my upper lungs. With each inhale, my upper lungs are fully expanding, and I'm enjoying a new increase in energy, clarity, memory, verbal and physical skills, being centered, and of course, inner awareness. In less than a month, it's natural to breathe only into my upper lungs.

Breathing *only* into the middle section of my lungs, takes a little less than a week. Next, I practice breathing *only* into my lower lungs. With each breath I'm aware of my abdomen moving in and out, which is cultivating the chi in my *tan tien or sea of chi* located below the navel. In a few days, it's natural to breathe *only* into the lower section of my lungs.

My next step is to own the complete breath, connecting my full breath into my lower, middle, and upper lungs. In less than a week, the complete breath is natural, and *my inner awareness is enhanced and deepened far greater than doing any and all external martial art forms.* I'm now aware of my inner world of organs: lungs, heart, stomach, and also muscles etc. in ways I haven't experienced. Each time I practice my complete breath, my entire body is being nourished; my abdomen and internal organs receive a gentle massage which cultivates my chi. I practice or play with various breathing patterns while doing the complete breath and postures, and again this cultivates my chi and greatly increases my inner awareness. With the new levels of inner awareness, I'm experiencing a significant improvement in my inner and outer focus, energy level, clarity, memory, verbal and physical skills, being centered, and living more in the now.

Even though I own the 4 Levels of Breathing, the thought of meditating still feels completely overwhelming. Rather than focusing on how I feel, how much I have to do, and how long it will take to own meditation, I decide to change my mind-set. I begin coaching myself – big time. Before I meditate, I proclaim, *"It's Easy* to own meditation. *It's Easy* to keep delving deeper into my #1 brain healing technique; my inner awareness training. *I need to keep having faith in myself; I will succeed in owning meditation, and it will help me delve deeper into my inner awareness training."*

Day after day, I practice my precious inner awareness training while meditating. *After a few months of training, I'm shocked – meditating is natural; I feel as though I was born to meditate and do the internal martial arts. I laugh. I've come a long way from being completely skeptical to owning meditation. The answer is inside- my inner awareness training.*

The benefits from meditation, the internal martial arts, and chi are outstanding: I'm calmer, more centered, clearer, have more memory, energy, strength, my verbal and physical skills have improved, and I need less sleep. **The best part of meditation, internal martial arts, and chi is each time I practice them, I experience something new with my precious inner awareness training.**

It's only been about a year and a half since I started Phase I of my brain healing training. Although I am no longer light years away from where I was pre-TBI, my brain is far from completely healed. On the other hand, I no longer think of meditation as wimpy. I also continue to strongly sense I need to pursue the paths of meditation, the internal martial arts, and chi in order to delve deeper into my inner awareness training. But, I still don't know if they are powerful enough to break through the prison in my brain.

My test to 1st Degree Black Belt is right around the corner. With my new levels of inner awareness, energy, etc., my preparations are a little easier, yet it takes a lot of my time and effort to train for my test. I decide to continue working diligently on my testing forms. Compared to my fellow testing students, who are excellent martial artists, I have much work ahead. I am really looking forward to testing to 1st Degree Black Belt.

15

A BELT AND A
PIECE OF PAPER
ANOTHER TRAIL
ENDS
APRIL 1995

Another dream has come true; I am a 1st Degree Black Belt! What an accomplishment for anyone, but for a person with a TBI this is beyond awesome! I love that I continue achieving more than anyone else thought was possible, and that so many "no's and never's" are now in the past. Although there are more to overcome, one day I will triumph over all of them and be better than before the TBI.

Dad and I plan a trip throughout the West, including Yellowstone National Park. I will drive from Boulder, Colorado to Billings, Montana about 550 miles in my big ole ass truck with my dog Maja. Dad will fly from Boston to Billings, and I'll pick him up at the airport. I organize my travel plans, and also our plans after Dad arrives in Billings. Next, I prepare my big ole ass truck and stock up on supplies. I am really looking forward to seeing the sights in Wyoming and Montana before Dad arrives at the airport.

I leave Boulder excited for my road trip; the landscape is green and the wildflowers are gorgeous. Shortly after I cross the Wyoming border, especially after leaving the Cheyenne area, the landscape dramatically changes. It's completely barren, except for the humongous snow fences. I have never seen such tall and long fences; they certainly know how to make snow fences. The monotony is broken up by the rare sightings of horses, cattle, pronghorn, or other animals. But, I get the willies when I see vultures circling overhead. Beforehand, I decided to do my trip in two days, stopping off in Casper, Wyoming to see the sights. The next day, I leave Casper a little disappointed.

About 150 miles later, the landscape becomes livelier. I cross the border into Montana, and the stunning mountains and Crow Indian Reservation beckons me to stop. I decide to keep driving to Billings in order to get everything squared away before picking up Dad in the morning. With the mountains behind me, I see a sight which I've heard about, but have never experienced. The Big Sky of Montana! It feels like I can reach out my truck window and touch this magnificent blue sky! A few miles later, I am in awe, as I watch a breathtaking, small, enclosed rain storm!

Up ahead is a road sign, there's a few more exits till I get to Billings, which gives me time to take stock of my brain healing journey. After I left rehab and Northeastern University, I wasn't capable of driving from Boulder, Colorado to Billings Montana by myself; now it is relatively easy. I absolutely cherish having more energy, being physically strong, and mentally clearer. I'm enjoying the living daylights out my life, and I am so hopeful. I know I'm going to continue making great strides and soon be better than before the TBI.

I enter Billings and find a nice park for Maja the wonder pup and myself to stretch our legs. I like giving people and animals nicknames; most people seem to like it. Next, I get squared away at the inn, refuel the truck, and explore Billings and the surrounding area for a few hours. Later, I have a great meal, and as usual, when my head hits the pillow, I sleep like a baby.

The next morning, I wake up refreshed and take Maja to a nearby park for her walk and my A.M. workout. When I finish my brain healing training, we take a nice walk around the park; the flowers and grass are beautiful. Up ahead is a pond with a wide array of noisy ducks, geese, and other waterfowl. This place is dog heaven and Maja is going nuts; thankfully, she's on a leash.

A few hours later I pick up Dad at the airport. The first place we visit is Little Big Horn Battlefield National Monument. Inside the visitor center we read about the battle, look at the maps, and drawings. About halfway through, Dad walks up to me and quietly says. "Custer wasn't the sharpest cornflake in the bowl." We laugh.

A few minutes later, a National Park Ranger walks in and announces the tour will be starting shortly. The ranger talks about the battle of Little Big Horn, and uses the words arrogant and stupid to describe Custer. Later, Dad and I take our own tour of the battlefield, and it's obvious the park ranger was being very polite when he described Custer.

For dinner we go to a local steak house in downtown Billings which we've heard is really good. The hostess seats us at a table, and we order our meal. While waiting, we observe a most interesting sight. A cowboy walks by all dressed up and sits at a table, but no one brings him a menu. He looks so content; I sense he's at peace with himself and the world. A minute later the waitress brings him a beer, and a few minutes later she brings his steak dinner with all the fixings. Dad and I look at each other, and we ask our waitress what just happened. She tells us, "Every Saturday night, he comes in, sits at the same table, has a beer, and a steak dinner. He'll pay his bill and goes dancing at the Grange Hall. At 10 P.M. he'll head back to the ranch so he can be on the range in the morning. He does this every Saturday night."

The next morning, Dad and I leave Billings and head west. We take turns driving so we can enjoy the gorgeous scenery. For lunch we have a great meal and meet more wonderful people. Everywhere we go, we meet the friendly people of Montana. We stop in Bozeman to visit the Museum of the Rockies which has a collection of dinosaur fossils and a great exhibit of Native American history. Bozeman, like the rest of Montana, is stunning.

The next day we enter Yellowstone National Park, and we marvel at all the breathtaking beauty. One moment, there's a spectacular waterfall diving into a crystal clear lake with rainbows leaping out of the billowing mist. A few miles later, there's a buffalo herd twenty yards away from the truck grazing on the thick emerald green grass. Up ahead is the Yellowstone River gently and gracefully meandering through the grassland; it's easy to sense the tremendous power of this majestic river.

We continue our exploration and the park changes dramatically. A major fire has destroyed a vast area. Most of mountains are marred with blackened tree trunks; however, a few mountains have come through unscathed. The park ranger explains that although the fire damage was massive, sprouting from the scarred earth are the most beautiful flowers and vegetation which no one has seen. The botanists are naming all these new plants. If there wasn't a fire, this spectacular new flora wouldn't have been discovered. This experience reminds me that with every challenge great or small, there are *always* huge positive and healthy breakthroughs and successes as long as I am open, look for, and purposefully work for positive and healthy changes.

We visit the different sights throughout Yellowstone and spend the night near a waterfall which lulls me to sleep. The next day we continue exploring this magnificent National Park and later drive through Grand Teton National Park, the Wind River Indian Reservation, and spend the night in Lander, Wyoming. We eat at a favorite local steak house and Dad has "the best steak ever." In the morning, while heading south back to Boulder, Dad is already making plans for our next trip. He has to go back to that steakhouse to get the six course 2 lb steak with all the fixings for $15.99.

After a few hours, Dad pulls up to a four-way stop sign in the middle of nowhere. There hasn't been a person, a house, or even an animal for over an hour. To our right, sitting on top of this enormous snow fence are two huge vultures staring at us. Dad and I give each other the look of 'let's get the heck out of here' and we're off like a shot. A few minutes later, these gorgeous mountains seem to sprout up; they look like someone has painted them. A sign up ahead tells us these are the "Painted Mountains," and Dad gets nostalgic. When he was a kid, he saw these mountains in the western movies, but he didn't think he would ever see them in real life.

When Dad's ready, we get back on the road. A few miles later, I become aware that I'm unsettled inside. I've been driving for five days, but part of yesterday, and most of today, I haven't been able to do my share of the driving. I love to drive, yet I haven't had the energy to drive. I know Dad doesn't mind driving. In fact, he loves to drive, especially my big ole ass truck. But, it really bothers me that I'm not able to pull my weight.

I pull my old cowboy hat over my eyes and sink into the seat. Although I've made great strides and have accomplished so many things the professionals said I could never, ever do. I am still imprisoned in the thick, blurry glass wall in my brain, and now, I don't have the energy to drive. I sigh. I'm not where I want to be, but gratefully I'm not where I used to be.

We get back to Boulder and spend some time in Colorado. After I drop Dad off at the airport, I take a more thorough stock of my brain healing journey. I've improved as a whole, and it's been a refreshing change to be productive, including earning my 1st Degree Black Belt. But, *I've hit a dead end. Long before I attained my Black Belt, the external martial arts utterly failed at improving my precious inner awareness training. I didn't think it was possible, but there is a finite limit to deepening my inner awareness with external martial arts, or any external movements like hiking, dancing, yoga, basketball, golf, etc.*

Finally, I accept my precious energy is being drained, and not replenished by the external movements. I've stayed on this external, dead-end path way too long because I didn't know what else to do. I was also having fun, I love the camaraderie with my workout buddies and other students at the school; it truly is special.

Next, I face the harshest reality of all. The idea of fixing my busted brain with a Black Belt makes about as much sense as going to college to get a degree; it feels like I'm rubbing salt into an open wound. I've gotten way off-track and lost my way. The prison in my brain is completely intact, and in my minds-eye, I'm still climbing in what I hope is upward in the dark, dank never-ending hole. Although I am immensely grateful for all the exceptional progress, there is much work ahead. I need to discover a new trail – technique to delve deeper into my precious inner awareness training. On the plus side, I wonder what good will come out of this misstep.

JUST TRUST
MID-AUTUMN
1995

For the past six months, I've been doing a lot more chi kung postures, tai chi forms, meditation, and other internal martial arts; it is now so easy to delve deeper into my precious inner awareness training. Though my inner compass is back on course, I still have enormous doubts about the power of chi and the internal arts. There's another reason I'm hesitant to dive into the internal martial arts. If I change focus, I may lose the companionship of my workout buddies at school; they pretty much only practice the external martial arts. But, if I just do the external martial arts or anything external, I'll get stuck and head backwards.

In any journey, it's good to be flexible and open. Immediately, I have a huge gut sense to keep persevering, be open, and trust the next right step will reveal itself. I reflect that the only thing that's helping me to delve deeper into my precious inner awareness training is meditation, chi kung postures, tai chi forms, and other internal martial arts. I decide to take a leap of faith, and give all of them my absolute best effort without bias.

Step by step, I practice and am flabbergasted at how simple and easy it is to understand, experience, and do the internal martial arts by utilizing my inner awareness training. I am thriving! The more I delve deeper into my inner awareness training while doing the internal forms, the wider the door opens to the internal martial art. The flow of chi moving inside me as I practice is extraordinary. My memory, verbal and physical skills, and energy are off the charts awesome. Until I come, face to face, with the Chen Tai Chi form.

Chen is an enormous form and has numerous "fa ching," or explosive chi energy strikes throughout the form. I listen carefully to students, with intact brains, say over and over again; Chen is too hard, too long, too complicated, too much work, and they're not going to practice the form. I don't understand their logic and I'm glad I don't. If you write notes and practice Chen, you'll own the form. Instead of focusing on what other people are saying and not doing, I consciously change my mind-set. "If I can own Chen Tai Chi – my brain can do anything. I will own Chen Tai Chi, and own it so well that I can *easily* teach it to others." Owning Chen will be my biggest task yet, and the decision to set my sights high puts a huge smile on my face.

I listen to my audio recordings of Chen Tai Chi and write, then re-write my notes. I also ask two upper Black Belts for a copy of their notes. Though I'm grateful for their notes, and they somewhat help, it's true what they say; every person's notes make sense only to them.

With enthusiasm, I practice Chen diligently while clarifying my notes, whittling them down to 11 power packed pages. In the beginning, I precisely audio record my notes; then, listen to them while doing the form which makes it easier to learn this massive form. To others this might seem like an enormous amount of work, but it isn't work – this is play. Rather quickly, I stop using the audio recording and notes, and practice the form *on my own*, and my improvements are far beyond exceptional.

Chen is generating a ripple effect, deepening my inner awareness and mindfulness, enhancing my ability to relax and root, while increasing my memory, energy, mental, verbal, and physical abilities. Again, each time I do Chen and other tai chi forms, meditation, chi kung postures, and my other internal martial art forms, **I am aware of something new in my precious inner awareness training, which greatly improves my inner, then outer focus in the foreign outside** world. I get the sense there will *always* be something new to experience and be aware of while doing my inner awareness training.

Adding Chen to all my other simultaneous brain healing techniques is helping me tap into deeper and deeper levels of inner awareness. I've grown far beyond muscles and joints. Now, I am aware of the subtle changes of chi in a global way from the inside out. I am also thoroughly enjoying the biggest increase in my chi, mental clarity, energy level, and of course my precious inner awareness training. There's something about owning the Chen Tai Chi form which has created a metamorphosis in my brain healing training and journey.

Deep in my gut, I know I'm going to need a heck of a lot more chi to break through the thick, blurry glass prison in my brain. I decide to increase my practice of meditation, chi kung postures, tai chi forms, and all the internal martial art forms. Although my progress continues to be absolutely remarkable, I keep coming face to face with my quandary. Do I move forward, or do I stay with my workout buddies at the school? It's time to make a decision.

16

A NEW DIRECTION
FEBRUARY 1996

I decide to make a leap of faith and blaze a new path in my brain healing journey. From now on, my whole focus is on meditating, chi kung postures, tai chi forms, and the other internal martial arts in order to delve deeper into my precious inner awareness training and to cultivate as much chi as possible. I have accepted that *any* outside method is *not* the answer to the inner problem of TBI. *The solution must come from inside.* I'm grateful for the solid foundation of, step by step, being aware of how my inner body responds to people and situations in the foreign outside world and being aware of my muscles, joints, etc., all of this was vital preparation for my next right path. The external martial arts and testing to the upper Black Belt levels are now a low priority. I record this momentous decision, because I always want to remember when I changed directions.

Internal Work
February 1996

Around my home, I put up "Internal Martial Art" signs to remind me of the importance of practicing everyday. There's a saying for internal work: if you miss a day, you lose three days of training. Miss a week, lose a month. Miss a month, lose a year. In my gut, I absolutely know that it's vital to be consistent in my inner awareness and internal martial art training in order to succeed in completely healing my brain. I set my goal: *everyday* I will do my internal training.

For the first month I do well, training before breakfast in order not to interrupt my digestion. My training is easy as long as I focus on delving deeper into my inner awareness. The challenge is getting started in the morning. Many mornings I'd rather be sleeping in, having breakfast, etc. Each time I want to do something else. I remind myself that shortly after I start, I'll experience the wonderful peaceful, energetic sensation of chi, which is now lasting about half an hour after I finish my training.

Day after day, I practice and the more days I compile – my inner awareness deepens to whole new levels, and my chi continues to be invigorated. It's very easy to be aware of my chi being developed during meditation, and I receive my confirmation when I practice my chi kung postures. My fingers are full of chi. Inside it feels like my fingers are big sausages; they feel really good, yet on the outside my fingers look and move normally. The benefits from my new training are phenomenal: *I have more energy, my thinking is a little clearer and faster, and I'm speaking quicker. I'm also able to remember longer forms and other information more easily.*

In March, month two, I miss two separate days of training. If I keep missing a day here and a day there, I'll never figure a way to completely heal my brain. Rather than kicking my butt, which would be a serious waste of time and energy, I decide to grow from this misstep. An analogy helps put everything into perspective.

I love good food, but it doesn't make sense not to eat for a day or two, or even a week, and then try to make it all up in one sitting. My training is as essential as food and water. Instead of practicing when I feel like it or when I think it's a good idea; I will practice my internal martial art training every day, no matter how I feel and no matter what's going on. I add a new motto to my brain healing journey: *"One brain healing training means I am one step closer to liberating myself from the TBI and being reconnected."*

Day after day I train, and weeks turn into months. Step by step, my inner awareness deepens and my invigorated chi has fully expanded into my hands, lower arms and elbows, and is just a little bit into my upper arms. In addition, the invigorating, peaceful sensation of chi is now lasting several hours after I train. Tapping into my chi has improved my inner and outer focus, and I am thoroughly enjoying a new level of energy and clarity, and I need less sleep. In addition, it's even easier to own and practice my forms, and to do *all* my activities even better. **What is shocking and off the charts awesome is now *all* my improvements: mentally, physically, verbally, energy level, etc. are happening at the same exceptional rate, not at the old three-tiered rate!**

I cherish each opportunity to do *all* my training and laugh at my former prejudices about meditation, chi, and the internal martial arts. Meditation is invigorating, healing, soothing, peaceful, and a pure joy. However, there are mornings when I still don't feel like working out. To get me out of bed I say to myself; Get going Cathy. In a few minutes you will be feeling really good. Before you know it, you're A.M. workout will be done and you'll be feeling even better! I get up and a few minutes after I start training; I feel awesome! As always I share with my workout buddies and friends at the school the ease of doing the internal martial arts. My hope is they'll start doing more of the internal martial arts, but their minds are made up. The vast majority of my friends are working on their next belt level. I accept their decisions and keep moving forward. I sense a great discovery is on the horizon.

17

A GIANT LEAP FORWARD - MY FIRST INTERNAL CONNECTION

The key to moving or opening to my next level is the 3 Day Inner Awareness Training to my Tan Tien or sea of chi. The tan tien is located below my navel; it's where the chi is stored. For three days, I need to be aware and connected to my tan tien: morning, noon, and night, eating, reading, writing, training, and even going to sleep. But the thought of being aware and connected to my tan tien for a solid three days with a busted brain is overwhelming. I believe this would be an arduous task for people with intact brains.

How the heck am I going to be aware and connected to my tan tien for three days with a TBI? What happens if I fail? What happens if I succeed? What do I do when I lose my inner awareness and connection? Will I have to go back to square one? I become aware that my shoulders are hunching in and my spirit is beginning to drag. Before I'm even out of the gate, the doubts are trying to set up housekeeping. Flashing before my eyes are people going on and on about all the things they can't do and how everything is too hard or impossible. Am I going to be a "want to, want to" and keep feeding the doubts; a dressed up version of fear? *No! I am going to take everything one moment at a time, then one day at a time, and I will do everything to the best of my ability. It's Easy to own the 3 Day Inner Awareness Training to my Tan Tien.*

I place many "T.T." tan tien signs around my home; they're a reminder to stay focused on the task of "looking within" or "Nei Se." To give me the best opportunity for success, I make a conscious effort to keep my surroundings calm and quiet. Equally important is the absolute necessity to be safe, for example driving a vehicle, cooking, etc. I've chosen a time that's most favorable for me, for some people a long calm weekend or a quiet vacation works best.

Day One – I wake up and the first thing I see is my "T.T." sign. I smile, and become aware and connected to my tan tien while placing the tip of my middle finger directly on my tan tien acupuncture point. I've read that some people use a small, sharp stone or thorn holding it in place with a belt over the tan tien to help them focus. Intentionally causing pain to be aware and connected is nuts; it is a backwards approach. I know how I work; I flourish in positive, healthy, and fun environments, and this is the atmosphere I have consciously created.

I breathe deeply while slightly wiggling my fingertip, and say, *"It's Easy* to be aware and connected to my tan tien." After a few seconds, my inner awareness and connection is stronger. I remove my finger, get up, pray, and prepare for my regular morning brain healing training: meditation, chi kung postures, and tai chi. In the middle of my workout I realize I'm not aware and connected in my tan tien. Rather than berate myself, I calmly become aware and reconnected. I am very delighted that during my morning training, I only have to refocus a few more times.

I finish my morning training and begin my daily activities while continuing to intentionally be aware and connected to my tan tien. Mid-morning, I'm in the kitchen looking for a snack and realize I've lost my inner connection. Gently, I become aware and reconnect to my tan tien.

At lunchtime, I take stock of my progress. Before I started the 3 Day Inner Awareness Training to my Tan Tien, I thought I'd have to reconnect to my tan tien all the time. However, it's only been about one to three times per hour. I'm not sure why it's been rather easy, until I realize that I've completely owned each step in my inner awareness and brain healing training before I moved on to my next right step. This great foundation and work ethic is two of the reasons I am thriving.

The rest of the afternoon and evening, I continue my training, and I am in awe of the results! I've been able to stay aware and connected to my tan tien more than I ever thought I could! I've also had to readjust my internal clock because I've taken another major step towards the foreign outside world. Although I don't know how many more steps there are before I am in sync with the foreign outside world; it no longer matters because I continue moving in the right direction – home.

While getting ready to sleep, I am aware of a great increase in clarity and energy, yet I am calm and centered. Once again, it's like my brain has been waiting for me to be aware and connected to my inner body, more precisely, to my tan tien. I am extraordinarily grateful – the 3 Day Inner Awareness Training is light years ahead of any other work I've ever done. Before going to sleep, I place the tip of my finger on my tan tien. I smile; I'm already aware and connected to my tan tien. I breathe, relax, and remove my finger, and go to sleep very hopeful.

Day Two – I wake up feeling even more centered and *in* my body than I have since the accident. Before I get out of bed I place my fingertip on my tan tien, breathe, and become more aware and connected to my tan tien. I have a great workout, and later that morning, I have an *Ah ha, knock my socks off moment. Being aware and connected to my tan tien is so much easier than it was on day one. I've had to refocus a lot less, and all my inner and outer abilities have been elevated to whole new levels. For a little over one day's worth of work, these are beyond remarkable results.*

With an extra spring in my step, I continue being aware and connected to my tan tien while doing all my brain healing trainings and all my daily activities. I have a phenomenal day, and before going to sleep I place my fingertip to my tan tien, breathe and relax. I remove my finger, and in a few moments, I am fast asleep. My precious inner awareness training is an extraordinary technique that keeps on giving.

Day Three – I wake up feeling more like the real me. My heart is filled with gratitude; I am even more aware and connected to my tan tien. I have so much energy, clarity, and I am more centered than day two. Next, I think about all the things I want to do and will accomplish today.

I have an awesome A.M. workout, morning, and lunch, and I rarely had to refocus to my tan tien. In the middle of the afternoon, I realize I am not aware and connected to my tan tien. **I start to move my finger but stop. I am stunned. I am already aware and connected to my tan tien without having to consciously focus to it! In less than three days, it is completely natural to be aware and connected to my tan tien! Many times throughout the day I think I have lost my focus, yet I am still naturally aware and connected to my tan tien. What seemed like an overwhelming task was so much easier and simpler than I thought.**

Pulsating in my tan tien is warmth; a wonderful sense of vibrant energy – life which is my confirmation; I have made my first internal connection! I have so much energy from my chi that I need to release and balance it, but I do not want to. I know I need to cultivate more chi not less, because I am going to need all the power I can muster to break through

the prison in my brain. On my next appointment with Yao, the acupuncturist, I receive another confirmation; she too experiences my invigorated chi.

I have a huge gut sense that I have crossed a mammoth junction in my brain healing journey. The 3 Day Inner Awareness Training to my Tan Tien was easier and simpler than I thought it would be, and everything in my brain healing training and life is easier and more fruitful. There is a noticeable release of pain from the 10" icicle in my left inner eye socket. However, when I get extra tired late at night, the pain returns; though, the level of pain pales in comparison to what I've had to endure for years. Although the thick, blurry glass wall is completely intact, it doesn't bother me because the pace and progress of my brain healing journey continues to increase at an astonishing rate – even for me. Also the climb in the never-ending hole in my mind's eye has become easier.

In addition, there are other benefits to naturally being aware and connected to my tan tien which I did not expect. It's easy to be aware of or know where people's center is located, and it's shocking how few people are in their tan tien. This is very noticeable when people are taking legal or illegal drugs or substances that affect the brain. Their center is not even within their body; it's above their head. Here is an example. As soon as I see a friend of mine, who is an excellent martial artist and a great human being, I know something's wrong. I ask her what's up. She tells me her allergies have kicked in. My next question gets right to the point. What are you on because you are always in your tan tien? But now, your center is about six inches above your head. She tells me she's taken some over the counter allergy medicine which is messing her up. She feels cloudy and can't think right. A little later, she tells me she's going home to get some sleep. I wish her well; hopefully, in the morning, she will feel like herself.

Being aware of the location of a persons center is a valuable tool during tai chi blindfold sparring, which develops sensitivity, awareness, and intention: first, within the practitioner; second, with the opponents intent of when and where they're going to strike, deflect, or move; and third, with the practitioners surroundings. One of the keys to tai chi blindfold sparring is to be soft and relaxed; using force only strokes the ego which ultimately defeats the practitioner.

There is also an interesting saying for tai chi sparring; *follow and get there first*. This means that by being aware of the opponent's intent, the practitioner can arrive first and neutralize a strike or take advantage of a deflection. Owning this skill is a huge advantage; however, for me to rise to this level will take a great deal of work. *With time and effort, my inner awareness training will help me transform the tool of "follow and get there first" into a brain healing technique; to be clear this technique will have nothing to do with tai chi sparring. In the future, this brain technique will be a crucial; although, a small tool that will help me at different times in my brain healing journey.*

My first step in "follow and get there first" is to be aware of my own intent or thinking before I move, strike, deflect, and stop, while practicing my internal forms, tai chi blindfold sparring, and also in my daily activities. My hope is that being aware of my thinking before I move etc. will help me delve deeper into my precious inner awareness training. I begin a tai chi form, and after a few moves, I am surprised at how unaware I am of my thinking. Day after day, I practice diligently, and slowly, very slowly, I begin to be aware of my thinking – intent before I move, etc.

18

LASER FOCUS

The solution to TBI must be chi – it has too be! I need to cultivate as much chi as possible and make it strong enough to break through the prison in my brain. Immediately, I get a very strong gut sense that my training and chi *always* needs to be balanced. I consider the Yin Yang principle; two complementary energies that are always in a state of change while maintaining balance and harmony. Everything in life is continuously moving and changing and needs to be balanced. But, the Yin Yang principle does not apply to me, because I have a TBI and my energy level is still below where it was pre-TBI. I need *more* chi. I do not need to balance my chi. Besides I am further along the internal martial art path than most people, I can definitely handle a huge increase in chi. With a laser focus, I practice cultivating and enhancing my chi, and oh yeah, developing more inner awareness. The more I train, the more chi I develop, and it is exhilarating. Imagine a person with a busted brain using the word exhilarating to describe her energy!

The warmth of summer 1996, sparks me to increase my brain healing training even more. *Now, I am naturally meditating in my daily life: preparing meals, washing the dishes, gardening, hiking with the dog, doing my forms, classes, reading, etc. Life is great, my energy level is off the charts, my thinking is clearer, and I am moving and rooting better. Although I continue to strongly sense that I need to, step by step, deepen my inner awareness, I focus on cultivating more chi.*

When I am specifically practicing meditation, I no longer use a timer and every aspect of basic meditation is second nature. I prefer two postures: standing and sitting. In the sitting posture or tailor style, I am aware that my body leans to the right and my head tilts even further to the right. Since the accident my brain has always felt extra heavy, but I did not know I was leaning to my right side. Other than the TBI, I am in excellent health. Is my body and head leaning to the right because the vast majority of damage is to my left temporal lobe? Although I believe the reason I am leaning to right is a direct result of the TBI, I do not know for sure. However, now that I understand the problem (leaning to my right side); it will be easier to find then apply the solution. My next sitting meditation I add on the task of correcting my posture, or as I like to put it, compensating for my heavy head. Rather quickly, it becomes second nature to be aware and correct my posture.

Next, I apply having good posture while practicing my chi kung postures, tai chi, other forms, and daily life, etc. However, I face an unusual hurdle when I practice standing on one foot, leaping, and landing on one foot. It's like I need to do all these calculations to counterbalance my heavy head with the rest of my body. Could this be the reason why I had, and have more difficulty moving and doing my martial art forms than people with intact brains? I do not know. To offset this very different challenge, I go back to what has always worked – my inner awareness training. Slowly, very slowly my balance improves, but it is no where near not where I want it to be.

On a positive note, the wonderful sensation of chi from my early morning workout is lasting into the afternoon, and the chi has expanded through my upper arms, into my chest and upper back. Being aware, connected to, and following the living, powerful, pliable energy of chi is extraordinary as it simultaneously is strengthening and relaxing my muscles and body, and of course, deepening my inner awareness. Now, when I do my chi kung postures, I am using more of my chi to hold up and move my arms rather than 100% of my muscles. Even my wrist is stronger, has more range of motion, and is less painful. I am also experiencing what I can only describe as internal growing pains, which are similar to the growing pains I had as a teenager. But, these internal growing pains are different, they are not as painful, and they feel like my whole body is adjusting to the increase in chi and the way it moves. My breathing is also deeper and fuller which is cultivating more chi and more internal growing pains. Another outstanding benefit of my brain healing training is meeting new people. I like for people to get to know me as who I am – now. If it's appropriate, I explain about the TBI, but people are having a hard time believing that I ever had a TBI. At first I tried to convince people, but I've learned to take their doubts as a great compliment. I have come a long way and have made great strides. But, the prison in my brain constantly lets me know that I have more work ahead.

I decide to let go of my volunteer job at the riding center. I am very grateful for all the opportunities; however years ago, I learned everything I needed from horses for delving deeper into my inner awareness training. Now, it's time to cultivate a lot more chi.

19

A GENTLE
CAUTION THEN A
HUGE WARNING

With an extra spring in my step and huge smile on my face, I walk into Yao's acupuncture office. I tell her about the outstanding vitality of chi and how good I feel. Yao does her usual thorough examination and tells me I have *too much chi*. My first thought is she is daft. How can I have too much energy? I've got a TBI. Who's ever heard of a person with a TBI having too much energy? Not me.

Even though Yao is an M.D. in China, has studied with the best doctors in all of China, and is an excellent acupuncturist. I decide to disregard her advice because she does not know or understand what it's like to be imprisoned in the brain. How can she know? She has an intact brain. I'm not sure if people with intact brains will ever understand why I am working so hard to discover a solution to liberate myself so I can be reconnected. I don't know if people with intact brains will ever be able to comprehend what it's like to be completely disconnected from everything outside the prison in the brain, and I hope they will never, ever have to experience it for themselves. On the other hand, it's none of my business what anyone thinks, says, or does.

Yao asks me to cut back on my kung fu training. In my mind, I think she means external martial arts, and I reduce my external workouts. However, I continue making tremendous strides cultivating and enhancing my chi, and I am getting wonderful results. The improvements in the clarity of my thinking, speaking, and energy level lead me to cultivate more chi. Month after month, Yao advises me to decrease my kung fu workouts and I do, and my chi continues to greatly improve.

It's early February 1997, and I feel like I am entering a metamorphosis. For whatever reason, I do not want anything heavy or constricting on my head and body. My head is very hot, and it hurts to wear my old cowboy hat and baseball hats, and I stop wearing them. I am also wearing shorts or sweatpants with the legs pulled up above my knees, and I must always be barefoot inside my home. I do not know how to explain what I am experiencing, other than *the heat is being produced from inside me, not from the outside.*

Spring is right around the corner, and I feel like a car running on high idle that is stuck at a red light. I am full of energy but all jumpy inside. The wonderful sensation of chi is now a memory, and the great fog of TBI has returned and settled in thick again. My head feels so big and hot. But, I continue cultivating my chi because it is the only thing that has given me energy, and one day, I know I'm going to need all the power I can muster to break through the prison in my brain. Mostly, I keep building my chi because I don't know what else to do.

Mid-spring everything comes to a head, literally. While doing cat style push-ups I collapse face first onto the floor. More precisely, it feels like this overpowering energy is continuously driving my head not onto, but *into* the floor. I try to get up using my arms, but there is no up. Finally, I'm able to push myself up. My head feels like this huge super punch exploded up my spine and slammed full force into my brain. Everything begins to get back to normal, and I resume my cat style push ups. Wham! Once again, I am being face planted *into* the floor. I try to stand up, but there is no up. Slowly, I crawl on all fours to the wall, then try to pull myself up to sit or stand, but once again there is no up. I resign to sitting on the floor and leaning against the wall. What the heck just happened? Why am I so disorientated, and where did that super punch come from?

The next time I see Yao I get my answer, but I don't like it. I have developed "Rising Chi" or "Shang Chi," and I have to stop *all* my kung fu practice, internal and external. Then, she delivers the ultimate blow – I have to disperse *all* the chi I've developed until I am balanced. She tells me she knows how difficult it was to hear this news; it was extremely hard for her to tell me. Next, she asks me to talk with the instructors about the best way to deal with rising chi. I take a deep breath, look her right in the eye, and say, "They do not know what to do." Yao gets angry, not so much at me, but at the infuriating situation of poor teaching. Yao suggests I sit in my backyard in the grass to disperse my excess chi, and not to practice any kung fu, of any kind, for at least 2 – 3 months, maybe more. With my head hung low, I sit in her office completely dejected. That evening I go to the school and ask what can I do for rising chi. "What does Yao say?" The question does not surprise me. I decide to follow all of Yao's suggestions. The question of how I am going to completely heal my brain is temporally replaced with how the heck did I get so off-course, and what good is going to come from this misstep.

20

MISSTEPS - A NATURAL PART OF ANY JOURNEY SPRING 1997

Life is blossoming all around me, yet here I sit in the grass with my very sore head dispersing my precious chi. Day after day, and week after week, I feel motionless; my brain healing journey has come to a complete stop or so I think. When my inner balance begins to return, I search for where my thinking, decisions, and actions veered off-course. The story about a compass helps guide me. If a person starts a journey off by one degree, they could miss their destination by a thousand miles.

It's easy to see where I went off-course, and how my arrogance and immaturity drilled me into the floor. Consciously, I placed a higher priority on cultivating my chi than on my precious inner awareness training. I believed that because my inner awareness training and internal martial arts had come so easily to me that

I, the one who had made *all* this great progress, must be further along than other people. *I* didn't need the simple techniques that would have balanced me and my chi. *I* could handle the extra chi. **Well, La Ti Friggin Da.** In my mind I hear a mentor, "Cathy, stomp on your ego with both feet."

Two thoughts help square away my mind-set and get me on-course. First, out of every negative situation have come many positive, healthy experiences and transformations because I have learned to be open, to look for, and to purposefully work for them. Second, I wonder what good will come out of this experience.

Though Rising Chi is a very unpleasant experience, it is a wise and humble lesson. Firmly and permanently put in its place is being impatient, taking short cuts, and the idea that a person can't have too much chi, along with my arrogance and immaturity. I reflect on my brain healing insight; mistakes or missteps and techniques that do not work are a natural part of any journey. Rather than kicking my butt for this colossal misstep, I choose to continue healing from the rising chi. While I am balancing my chi, a series of events occurs which heals and releases me in ways I did not expect.

SHAKE, RATTLE, AND ROLLING FORWARD RELEASE FROM TRAUMA LATE MAY 1997

Another beautiful Colorado day and I am driving to my first appointment to release the traumas of the past. I park my truck and before going in, I take a moment to enjoy the stunning wildflowers on the surrounding hills, and to listen to the sound of water from the creek. The sights and smells of springtime help relax me. Though I am not sure how releasing the trauma works, I am hoping it will do a better job than all the years of traditional talking therapies.

The session begins with a brief explanation of the method, which is easy to understand. However, the words really take root and come alive when he verbally takes me through the technique. In a matter of a few minutes, he mentions my throat has turned bright red, but I am unaware. Now that I am paying attention I can feel my throat is constricted. There is a part of me that's bothered that I've been unaware, but there is an even bigger sense of relief. I have a gut sense; I need to trust.

Briefly, I relay the horrendous experiences of a few of the

brutal tortures, being strangled and almost dying, and the rapes by half-brother. When I finish speaking, he continues to verbally guide me. I begin to shiver, but I'm not cold. In a very gentle voice, he explains that what I am experiencing is natural. After a few minutes, the quivering travels throughout the trunk of my body, into my right arm, and out my hand. He relays this is a natural occurrence in animals, but we humans have forgotten how to release trauma.

The quivering stops, and for the first time in my life, I have a real sense of healing and release from the traumas of being strangled and almost dying. I have never experienced this depth of healing before. Though I feel slightly tired, I sense I have just taken another step towards freedom. I am surprised and delighted that my healing began from the inside out.

Swiftly, I ponder three points. First, my thinking is a bit faster and less congested. Removing the gunk of those traumas has calmed me. I do not have the same stuckness in my body and brain as I did before. Releasing these traumas has given me the relief I sought with alcohol, but never permanently received. Second, I think about the cancer that occurred in my neck and mouth. I no longer believe all the strangulations, torture, and abuse are a coincidence. Third, I think of all the time and money I have spent on talking therapies. The vast majority of time I left therapy feeling worse than when I went in. Talking stirred everything up, but never freed me. I ask why I didn't get the same kind of relief with the traditional talking therapies. He explains that when a person keeps talking and talking about a trauma; it can re-traumatize the person, rather than help. Although his answer surprises me, it makes perfect sense.

The hour session ends and he asks me to make an appointment with the neurologist who referred me; he will prescribe a medication. I am to open one capsule of Neurontin 100 mg and sprinkle the contents into a bottle of water 8 – 12 oz., and drink small sips throughout the day, and to do this for three to five days. I heed his advice.

Day one, of taking the prescription; my brain feels like it is trying to shift gears. Day two, my brain begins to slow down to a more normal speed. I am shocked. I did not know my brain was in hyper-mode since the TBI. I always thought my brain was in super, super slow motion. Now, I understand why I used to be completely exhausted by ten a.m. My brain was working at supersonic speed and it just plain wore out. Day three, I get the impression my brain has been on a rat wheel since the TBI. Now that the spinning wheel has slowed down enough for me to get off, I can finally move forward. Maybe this is another reason I have always felt stuck. I have been going round and round, watching where I wanted to go, and what I wanted to do, but I was getting nowhere fast. Could releasing the traumas be a solution to the TBI?

With each session I experience a release from trauma, an increase in healing, and a sense of being whole; it feels like I am being unconditionally loved from the inside. Also, I no longer have the intense need to be hyper-vigilant; to *always* protect myself from unknown dangers. The mental, physical, and emotional release from the traumas has given me freedom, peace, and connectedness which I have not felt since I was a little child.

Releasing trauma is a very short term therapy usually lasting between five to seven sessions. However, because of the severe level of trauma that I've experienced, I have more sessions. Although I am grateful for the healing and extraordinary results; releasing the traumas are *not a solution to TBI*. Life is funny. If I had not made the colossal misstep of cultivating too much chi, and not balancing myself and my training, I probably would have missed the tremendous opportunity to be healed from all the traumas. Hmm, a journey usually does not travel in a straight line. I always find it fascinating and comforting – when one door closes, another door or window opens.

FOUNDER, CEO, AND CHIEF BOTTLE WASHER MID-SUMMER 1997

With time on my hands, I am becoming even more social, and I love it. There are so many great events in the Boulder area. I am constantly asked if I went to the awesome concert, dance, or some other wonderful event. If I had known about the event, I would have gone. I realize if I am missing out on these great events, others must be too. I talk with the top leaders, heads of organizations, and other people in the area, and they too feel out of the loop. There's a lot of miscommunication going on here. Someone needs to create a place where people can easily get updated information of events on a regular basis. Immediately, I have a gut sense which shocks me. *I need to step up.* I need to start an info line; a free phone voice message with all the events in the area for gays, lesbians, the rest of the alphabet soup, and our straight allies. To my surprise, I soon become the Founder, CEO, and Chief Bottle Washer of the non-profit Boulder Gay Info Line.

Initially, I ask another person to record the voice message. *However, after two months, it's my job to record the power packed two minute voice message with all the events. At first, I am a little nervous.*

How can I say all this information and do it clearly with a busted brain? Out of pure necessity, I get over the jitters. Next, I train myself to clearly speak even faster in order to get all the events into a two minute voice message. Before I record the message, I clearly write the introduction, all the events, and thank the people for calling. It takes more than a few times to record the message.

The info line gets rave reviews. People are grateful to have a central location to find out what is happening in the community. Though there are a few people who think there are too many events and that *I am speaking way too fast.* They have to listen several times to get all the information. This is beyond hilarious. A couple of people, with intact brains, are trying to give me a hard time for speaking too fast. They do not have a clue that I could not speak a simple two to three word sentence after the TBI. I have come a long way and I love it!

I smile, and calmly explain that with the limited time and so many great events, I have to speak very quickly. I grin from ear to ear when I say I am from Massachusetts and this is my natural speaking pace. What I do not share is that I have a TBI and how much my verbal and all my skills have improved; far beyond what anyone else thought was possible. Yeaha!

The Boulder Gay Info Line is a one-person operation. In addition to recording the voice message, I attend events in Boulder County to publicize the info line, and also seek information about future events. I meet a lot of great people and make awesome connections in person and over the phone.

The first year, I ask different businesses to pay the monthly phone bill and they graciously help out. Each month I acknowledge the business that paid the phone bill. The second year, I will receive a grant. What a tremendous relief it will be to have the money to not only pay the phone bill, I will also print up business cards, magnets, flyers, and posters. With the additional advertising, the info line will get over 200 phone calls a month.

For many years, I will run the info line until a local organization takes over. Fortunately, years later, with the explosion of the internet, the Boulder Gay Info Line will become obsolete. A few people think I will be upset, but they do not know me. I am always looking for ways to improve on what works and to keep moving forward.

PHASE 2

NEW INTERNAL
CONNECTIONS

21

A MATURE
APPROACH
AUTUMN 1997

With new-found respect I resume my brain healing journey. I am profoundly grateful for the privilege of doing my healing training, and I do not take it lightly. I am no longer concerned with what's next, how much I have improved, and how quickly I will complete each task. I am certainly not focused on when I will liberate myself from the prison in my brain. I have complete trust that I will. From now on, I will be patient and methodically move forward. *Of the utmost importance is to always begin my brain healing training with the main purpose of delving deeper into my precious inner awareness training and balancing my self, my training, and my life.*

Patiently I daily meditate, practice chi kung postures, tai chi, other internal and external forms, and conditioning and stretching while being aware and connected to my tan tien which, of course, *all* of it deepens my precious inner awareness training. Rather quickly, the wonderful sensation of calm, centered chi returns and is lasting even longer into the afternoon. The chi has also permeated further and deeper into my body. I love delving deeper into my inner awareness training by being aware of how my chi is being cultivated, invigorated, moving, connecting, and working, which is helping me to be a little more in sync with my chi. Within weeks, all of my brain healing training has once again become effortless.

Almost another week passes, and I am again naturally meditating in daily life while being aware of my inner body, which means it's time to step up to a more advanced level of meditation. Thankfully, I have already completed the first requirement of advanced meditation; my basic meditation practice is completely natural to do. More importantly, I no longer have to focus on my inner awareness training while doing basic meditation. I also have a great head start in circulating my chi, because the chi flow always begins and ends in my tan tien, my first internal connection.

For advanced meditation, it is imperative to *mentally* cultivate, enhance, guide or direct my chi; I *must not* use my breath to do these actions. Again, people who are mentally unstable are not taught how to move or circulate chi because they could lose what little grasp of reality they have left. I have a gut sense the reason for not teaching these techniques to mentally unstable people will be revealed very shortly.

One of my goals for advanced meditation is to mentally circulate my chi throughout my body, breaking through one blockage at an acupuncture point and making one connection at a time. This is a slow, step by step process, and as always in my brain healing journey, each step must become second nature before moving on to the next level.

My first step is, of course, deepening my inner awareness. While meditating I will concentrate on experiences that are meaningful to me: happy memories, beautiful scenery, inspiring phrases, etc. My first wonderful memory is my Uncle Phil's magnificent garden. In sitting meditation posture, I innately switch my inner awareness to my tan tien. In my mind's eye, I see myself sitting in the backyard looking at a stunning red rose bush in full bloom. Step by step, my inner awareness naturally deepens by focusing to a single rose, a petal; then, a dew drop gently being held in perfect balance on a petal. The sunlight is creating a glistening rainbow on the dew drop and the colors are spectacular. Next, I utilize my other senses to fine tune my inner awareness; the sweet fragrance of the rose and the soft velvet of a petal calms and centers me, and of course, naturally deepens my inner awareness. Step by step, it's easy to increase the length of meditations and all my other brain healing training. Once again, I am thoroughly enjoying great improvements in all areas – simultaneously: cognitively, physically, verbally, chi, inner and outer focus, energy level, etc., and naturally my inner awareness. I am grateful that my progress is not at the old three-tiered rate.

I end my meditation, and in the future, will end all my meditations by returning my inner awareness to my tan tien to gather, store, and balance my chi, my self, and my training. I continue my brain healing training: practicing chi kung postures, tai chi, and other internal forms. When I finish working out, I balance and further ground myself by either doing punches in a horse stance, external forms, or going for a walk. As always, I wait 45 minutes before I go to the bathroom, eat, or sit down.

There is a surprising and wonderful benefit from all my progress; I want to work with wood again. But the thought of working with wood scares the living daylights out of me; I am afraid of getting hurt like I did with the TBI, maybe worse. Up until this moment, I did not know that I was afraid of working with wood. To shift my mind-set, I focus on the wonderful memories of working with wood. I thoroughly enjoyed the process of picking the right project, the types of wood, how I'd use the grain and sometimes even the knots to accentuate their beauty. I loved the pure satisfaction of using my hands to transform the rough wood into beautiful projects. Next, I think of future projects I want to design and build.

My mind-set changes again. All the crushing "no's and never's" are pounding in my head. "You will never, ever be able to work with wood again." "You will never be able to go to school." "You will never ever be able to do anything physical, ever again." "No, you will never be able to garden." I begin to panic. Arrgh, I have shifted my focus and allowed fear in.

I take a deep, long breath. Having courage is not the lack of fear or not feeling afraid. Courage is walking up and through the fear, and the vast majority of fears are not even real. I decide to take responsibility for my thinking and see the truth of the situation. Consciously, I switched my mind-set and started to feed and buy into the lies, or more precisely, other people's truths of *their* "no's and never's." I have already gone to school and did remarkably well. I have attained my 1st Degree Black Belt, and I am in better shape and more physically active than I was pre-TBI. My memory, energy level, physically, verbally, mentally, etc. has significantly improved. I have already had a great garden, and I drive my big ole ass truck where and when I want to.

With my thinking turned around, it's easy to see a solution. Maybe, if I gradually work with wood, it might be easier and even more enjoyable than before the TBI. I start a small project, but shortly after I begin, I stop. I have a gut sense not to push myself through this project or kick myself in the butt for stopping. Instead, I decide to have fun by getting familiar with my hand woodworking tools and arranging my tiny shop.

Before I pick up my block plane, one of my favorite hand tools, I naturally deepen my inner awareness and connect to my inner body. Next, I take my time setting the cutter, the cap iron, and lock everything in place. I rest the plane on its side so as not to nick or dull the blade. I choose a piece of scrap wood and place it in the bench clamp. Next, I pick up the plane and find a comfortable, solid stance while being relaxed and flexible. Using my whole body, I plane the wood. I am aware of familiar muscles, joints, etc., but there are slight differences in how they are moving and connecting. Simultaneously, I am fine-tuning the plane until the curl shavings flow smoothly out the throat of the plane. My heart is singing as I smell the sweet aroma of fresh wood and the sensation of shavings flowing over my hand. Each time I adjust my stance, shoulders, elbows, wrist, and root; my inner awareness naturally deepens. With everything aligned, my movements are flowing freely and as one. My inner awareness is now completely natural while planing the wood. Next, I safely deepen my inner awareness by closing my eyes. With each pass over the wood, I am more aware of how my inner and outer body is moving. I am also listening to the sound of the plane as it effortlessly glides over the wood; it is music to my ears. Being one with the plane reminds me of my inner awareness training.

Opening my eyes, I watch the curled shavings roll over my hand and land at my feet. My smile widens as I touch the planed surface; it's as smooth as glass. Closing my eyes, I run my fingers over the polished planed surface, then on the other side which is rough. I am aware of the small hills and valleys of the coarse wood. Being aware of both surfaces further develops my tactile sense, and more importantly, deepens my cherished inner awareness. I continue working, or as I like to say, *playing* with each hand tool; it feels I am like hanging out with old friends who I have not seen in years.

When I am comfortable with my hand tools, I pick up my circular saw. Before plugging it in, I take a minute to make sure I am squared away. Having respect for a woodworking tool, a brain healing technique, or any tool is crucial for success. Intentionally, I deepen my inner awareness while clamping a scrap piece of wood onto my workbench. Using a square, I clearly draw several lines across the wood. I put on my safety glasses, ear protection, and make sure my shoulder is dropped, wrist is aligned, and my elbow is braced against my side. I take a deep breath and start the circular saw. A huge smile comes over my face as I listen to the muffled whirl of the blade. After a few passes, I cut a nice straight line. *The real gift is the noise from the circular saw does not bother me at all!*

Rather than start a project, I create woodworking jigs, which in the future will make it easier to work on projects. Next, I shape the wooden handles on my martial art straight swords, broadswords, and spear etc. so they fit perfectly into my hands.

I show my workout buddies and other students at school my handy work explaining how I shaped them. A few of them tell me they are going home to fix theirs right away. I continue having fun working with wood and my tools, but I do not let it or anything else get in the way of my brain healing journey.

22

FINE TUNING THE
KEY
EARLY SPRING
1998

I am grateful for the solid foundation I have built, and that I 100% owned each technique before moving on to the next step. If I had not done *all* the work, I would not be ready for the next level in my precious inner awareness training. I will be *mentally* guiding or directing my chi from my tan tien through my body, to break through a lock and make a connection to the *ming men*, the life gate, near the kidneys.

Immediately, I am overwhelmed by the complex system of meridians and acupuncture points with their numbers, letters, and dots that crisscross the body. It looks like a badly drawn map. *To square away my mind-set, I decide to, as always, keep it simple and break everything down so it's easy to understand and apply.*

Meridians remind me of blood vessels in the body or electrical wires in a home. Meridians are hollow pathways or tubular channels, and the chi is the energy that flows in the meridians. Acupuncture points are where the chi comes near or to the surface. I think of acupuncture points as outlets in a home.

Next, I use a few analogies to help me understand all of this. When there is a blockage or lock in a meridian or acupuncture point, the chi flow is decreased or the flow completely stops creating an imbalance, pain, and or other problems. I think of a chi blockage, stagnation, or lock as a blocked artery in the body or a water hose that's bent. When there is a reduction in the flow of blood in an artery, a person can experience pain, difficulty breathing, and / or a loss of energy, etc. Bottom line, the person does not feel good. When the obstruction is removed in the artery or the hose is straightened the fluid gushes through and returns to its normal, healthy rate. There are several ways to release a chi blockage or lock. An acupuncturist uses acupuncture needles, acupressure, and / or herbs. But, these are external methods which are incapable of breaking through the prison in my brain.

To delve deeper into my inner awareness training, I will be utilizing advanced meditation to mentally break through a lock and make a connection which will allow the chi to flow. With my mind-set squared away, I am ready to meditate. I have a huge gut sense that something big is about to happen.

When I am calmly aware and connected in my tan tien, I guide my chi from my tan tien through my body to the ming men, the gate of life. To cultivate and strengthen the chi, I direct my chi to the tan tien; then, I guide the invigorated chi to the lock at the ming men. Each time I guide my chi between my tan tien and ming men, my inner awareness naturally deepens, and my chi gets stronger and more vibrant. It's rather easy to be aware of the chi building up and pushing on the lock at the ming men. **The chi pushing against the ming men reminds me of pushing against the thick, blurry glass wall in my brain. The significance of being aware and experiencing both; the lock**

on the ming men and the thick, blurry glass prison in my brain is beyond intriguing.

I deepen my inner awareness, which again invigorates my chi, and the lock at the ming men becomes slightly painful. *A very small crack appears on the lock and I visualize my chi like it's a sharp woodworking chisel and place it into the fracture. Within seconds the lock opens. There is a slight feeling of pain that quickly dissipates into a wonderful sensation of warmth, fullness, and vibrant pulsating chi. My ming men is whole and alive, and I've made my second internal connection! I have connected my tan tien and ming men!*

Now, it is time to have fun cleaning the pathway between my tan tien and ming men. My work becomes a *game of chi ping pong* which cleans up the debris in the pathway, and of course, naturally deepens my inner awareness, which enhances and increases the chi's velocity. Once I am proficient at guiding my chi back and forth between my tan tien and ming men, I have a most interesting experience, which in the future will help me enormously. **The chi transforms into a ball of light with a small tail which sort of looks like a comet. With daily practice my inner awareness improves significantly and my chi comet becomes fuller, brighter, and quicker. I am guiding my chi, and I am also ahead and following my chi. Following my chi comet reminds me of the saying for tai chi sticky hands sparring: follow and you get there first. The more I practice, the better I am able to guide and follow my chi which improves my inner awareness immensely. This is another momentous experience – I am easily guiding and following my chi, and I am doing it with a TBI!**

At the time I had no idea that by breaking through and connecting my tan tien to my ming men, cleaning up the pathway, and playing my game of chi ping pong that I had discovered the key to unlocking the prison in my brain. However, before I am ready to break through the thick, blurry glass wall – the lock in my brain, I will need to, step by step, fine tune my key of inner awareness.

MING MEN
PERIOD

A real-life benefit of opening and connecting my ming men is feeling good during my menstrual cycle. A few days before I begin my period, I consciously change my awareness from my tan tien to ming men (the gate of life). When I am almost through my period, I move my awareness to my tan tien until the next month. I am so used to feeling good during my period that when I forget to move my inner awareness before my cycle, it is quite obvious; I feel lousy. As soon as I move my inner awareness into my ming men, I feel better.

As always, I share with my fellow martial artists and friends what I have learned and experienced with chi and connecting my tan tien and ming men. They think it's so cool and interesting, but their ears really perk up and they lean in when I share the real-world results of feeling good during my menstrual cycle. Many women and men, inquiring for their girlfriends, wives, and mothers, ask how I opened and connected my tan tien and ming men. I explain the meditation technique and the foundation that it was built upon. Before each conversation ends, I ask them to let me know their results. Time after time, people walk up with a huge smile and share how they thought it was going to be very difficult and take a long period of time to move their inner awareness from their tan tien to ming men. They were pleasantly surprised how easy it was to apply this technique and how much it helped.

23

I AM THE HEALER
AND
THE ONE BEING
HEALED
SPRING 1998

My next right step is to *connect the two centerline meridians* in my upper body: the Governing and the Conception meridians. Looking at my acupuncture doll, I see the right side is in English and the left is in Chinese. Next, I examine acupuncture charts; I have only been able to find a few and they are not very good. Again, there is a vast system of meridian lines that crisscrosses the body, and the letters, numbers, and dots represent acupuncture points. Rather than be confounded and overwhelmed by how difficult it will be to understand this densely packed information, and the lack of, or the minimal instruction which has been taught extraordinarily complicatedly.

I consciously change my mind-set. *It's Easy* to connect the two centerline meridians in my upper body: the Governing and the Conception meridians which are called the Microcosmic Orbit or the Small Circle of Heaven. Again, I am not interested in arguing about the correct spelling and pronunciation of Chinese words or the different names used to describe techniques that would be a waste of time which will only take me off-course. My focus is to delve deeper into my precious inner awareness training and to balance my self, my training, and my life. I decide to simple call this step; *connecting the centerline meridians in my upper body.*

Eagerly, I use the acupuncture doll, charts, and my body to map the Governing meridian which rises up the midline of the back, neck, head, and ends at my upper gum. Next, I map the Conception meridian which descends along the front midline of the body. The two centerline meridians do not connect; there is a gap at the mouth. To connect the two centerline meridians in my upper body, I need to place the tip of my tongue, with a little saliva, on the roof of my mouth next to my teeth. *Now, it makes sense why my tongue needs to be in this position when I meditate and do my other internal martial art training. The tongue with a little saliva makes a connection or bridges the gap between the two centerline meridians and completes the circuit of chi.*

While mapping the acupuncture points in my body, I notice there are minor variations between the charts, my acupuncture doll, and my body. To precisely know where an acupuncture point is located in my body, I will need to personally experience each point using my inner awareness training. As always, intellectual knowledge is good, but it won't get the job done. I quickly think of the future, and that *when I teach my method in person, I will be very thorough and precise in my explanations of my inner awareness training, every brain healing technique, and my whole method.* However, if I wrote down my whole method it would take 1000's and 1000's of pages to explain all that I have and will do in my brain healing journey, but this would be incomplete, because *again, my method needs to be taught in person.*

Before meditating I again remind myself that my main goal is to always delve deeper into my inner awareness and to balance my self, my training, and my life. My meditation begins, and when I am calmly aware and connected in my tan tien, I consciously guide my chi from my tan tien to the fortified door of the first lock by the tip of the coccyx. Although the lock is more formidable than my ming men, it is a tremendous opportunity to deepen my inner awareness. *To break through the locks in the centerline meridians in my upper body*, I utilize the same technique that connected my ming men. Step by step, I purposefully deepen my inner awareness. A small fracture appears on the lock. I concentrate my inner awareness intensely into the crack which builds up my chi. Almost instantly the lock opens and my chi makes a connection. Again, I experience warmth, fullness, the vibration of life, and a new level of inner awareness, clarity, and energy.

The next lock in the centerline meridian in my upper body is the ming men. What's interesting is breaking through the lock by ascending upwards is much easier than going through the body. I believe it's easier because I have already broken through the bigger lock on the inner side of my ming men. I split my chi a little above my ming men; however, splitting my chi really isn't noticeable because the points are so close. Once I have broken through and made the connection, the chi returns to the centerline meridian.

So far, it's been rather simple and easy to follow the meridian, break through the locks and make the connections, and even doing a small split of my chi is much easier than I thought. Ahh, the more I practice, the more I improve at deepening my inner awareness.

The next real lock is the centerline point at my shoulder level which supposedly is difficult to get through, but it's rather easy to break through and make a connection. However, the lock where the neck joins the skull is much more impressive. This will be challenging for two reasons. First, there is a curve in the meridian. Second, I am farther away from my tan tien, my starting point where my chi is stored, cultivated, and invigorated. To square away my mind-set, I use the analogy of a rubber hose. The farther away an obstruction or the hose is bent (curve in the meridian) from the faucet (tan tien), the more water (chi) is needed to break through the lock. The key to breaking through locks that are farther away from my tan tien and that are curved is patience, and of course, deepening my inner awareness.

Initially, I am surprised how easy it is to move my chi such a long distance; I thought it would take an enormous amount of time. *Ahh, again time is irrelevant. What's most important is always deepening my inner awareness.* I break through the lock where the neck joins the skull, and again, the chi makes a connection and flows freely.

I follow the meridian to the pillow point, where my head hits the pillow. The next point is the top of my head, the crown point or the point of one hundred revelations, but this phrase is misleading. People who break through and connect to the crown point, then decide to stop at this point rather than move to the next point will have hallucinations which they believe are real, and they will be permanently stuck at this point. Now it makes sense why people who are mentally unstable are not taught how to circulate chi because they could lose what little grasp of reality they have left.

Before I begin meditating, I consciously make two decisions. First, after I have broken through the lock and have made the connection at the crown point, I will move without hesitation to my next acupuncture point. Second, if I do have illusions which draw me to stay at the crown point, I will ignore them. Because of the TBI, I know not take any chances; I need to be extra careful. I break through the crown point and feel the beginning pull of a delusion, but I do not focus on it. Instead, I easily move to the next point. After that I break through the point where the tip of my tongue touches the roof of my mouth connecting the Governing and Conception meridians, and I have a huge realization.

Once I mapped the meridians on my acupuncture doll, charts, and in my body. I needed to follow the meridian in my body until I reached a lock. I did not need to know the names of the meridians, the acupuncture points, where the blockages should occur. I simply needed to follow the trail until I reach a blockage, break through it, and make a connection.

Easily, I guide the chi down the midline of my chest and into my tan tien. In less than six weeks, I have connected the centerline meridians in my upper body into one meridian and – it was much easier and simpler than I thought.

Next, I clean the centerline meridian in my upper body of any gunk that is obstructing the flow of chi, just as I did between my tan tien and ming men. This clean up work, or more precisely play is a lot of fun, and once again, fine tunes and deepens my inner awareness. When my chi is circulating freely in the centerline meridian in my upper body; the chi's velocity is increased, which further enhances the vibrancy of my chi, and of course, deepens my inner awareness.

Guiding and following my bright, strong and fast chi comet is not only fun, it also improves my focus in the foreign outside world to whole new levels. I am more centered, clearer, have more energy, and the 10" icicle has completely melted. I have three huge gut senses. First, I have tapped into a crucial, but a foundational level of my brain healing training. Second, this entire step by step process will be essential in the rest of my brain healing journey. Third, each time I broke through a lock and made a connection, I sensed – I was one step closer to completely healing my brain. I have become the healer and the one being healed. I have heard and read about people who heal themselves by cultivating and invigorating their chi to break through locks, make connections, and clean up their meridians. However, I did not think I would be able to acquire these skills so easily and quickly. I am deeply humbled, honored, and extremely grateful. Inwardly, I enjoy this monumental milestone.

Before I can move forward in my brain healing journey, I need to figure out how to precisely circulate my chi throughout my body and into my limbs. But, there is very little information about this process and it is communicated in an extremely convoluted manner. There are no words that are strong enough to express how frustrating this is. While others see this as an obstacle, I see it as a positive challenge. I will find a solution. Again, I resolve that, in the future, I will precisely teach my brain healing method, in person, as I have blazed my journey. I will teach everything, especially my inner awareness training so it is easy to understand, apply and experience; and as always, I will continue to improve on what works. The next six months, my brain healing journey comes to a standstill or so I think.

In late October 1998, I start thinking about creating beautiful furniture and other projects. With time on my hands, I decide to design and build a table made with 5/4 cherry for the top and ash for the legs. To complete my project, I will need to buy a table saw, router with accessories, and other tools. I price the different hardware and tool outlets up and down the Front Range and the best deals are in two nearby cities.

Before I begin the table, I decide to become familiar with my new tools. Once again, I face the fear of getting hurt. Rather than buying into the lies and feeding the fears, I focus on: how much fun I will have, all the things I will learn, how much I will grow, and of course, the beautiful table I am about to build.

In early November 1998, I design and start building the table outside on the patio, because the garage is too small. For a large workbench, I use the custom sawhorses I made years ago and a piece of plywood for the top. Hauling all of the big equipment in and out of the garage: table saw, other tools, cords, saw horses, wood, especially at the end of the day gets old really quickly. When a sudden rain or snow storm comes in, I move fast and do not waste a step. To make my life easier, I build a ramp and a four-wheeled dolly to move the table saw and other big equipment in and out of the garage.

My heart is singing as I use my hands to transform the rough wood: cutting, routing, planing, gluing, and sanding. Best of all my head is not bothered by working outside in the brilliant sunshine or from the noise from the table saw, router, sanders, and other tools. As I apply the clear stain to the cherry table top, there is a tremendous transformation. The wood changes from a flat rust color to a stunning, luxurious, deep cherry. The beauty of the cherry will only get richer with age. In nine days I have taken a design from my head and used my hands to create a stunning table. A sense of pride wells up from deep within, and I take great satisfaction scratching off another "no and never."

My confidence has grown stronger, and I am more grounded, energized, balanced, and clearer in every area. Most importantly, my inner awareness training has again improved. Despite all of my accomplishments, the prison in my brain remains as strong, thick, and blurry as it was on day one, and in my mind's eye I continue climbing in utter darkness in the never-ending hole. None of that matters. I firmly believe that with my precious inner awareness training, a solution to the TBI must surely be around the corner.

24

EXPANDING MY
HORIZONS
LATE AUTUMN
1998

I need to find out why I am hesitant to move forward in my brain healing journey. First, I do not want to make another major mistake, which is natural, but that's not what's holding me back. I am tentative because the information about circulating the chi out of the torso and into the limbs is even more complicated and vague than it was to circulate the chi in the centerline meridian in my upper body. Supposedly, it is so difficult that few people even try. Maybe that's why many advanced meditation practices only go as far as circulating the chi in the centerline meridian in the upper body. Okay, I know I have been way too cautious, but trying to make good decisions with incomplete and obscure information is quite challenging and not in a good way. On the other hand, sometimes the worst thing to do is nothing. If I am going to keep moving forward, I need to put things into perspective.

Blazing my brain healing journey without a map has been a heck of a lot of fun, has produced remarkable results and positive transformations in all areas, and in a really good way has been quite a challenge. I have experienced and learned more about the human body than I ever thought I would, and I have done so much more physically and mentally than I ever thought I could. I have checked off many "no's and never's" and have far surpassed what the medical professionals or anyone else said was possible. On top of all that, I have a great head start in circulating my chi out of my torso and into my arms and legs because I have already connected the centerline meridian in my upper body.

Rising from deep within is an immense powerful drive and I begin coaching myself big time. *"It's Easy*, Cathy. Change your mind-set, expand your horizon, and go back to what has always worked. Continue delving deeper into your precious inner awareness training, balance yourself, and keep improving on what works." My task is simple; to break through one blockage and make one connection at a time. Immediately, I have another strong gut sense; it is just a matter of time and effort before I circulate my chi throughout my entire body. *It is not a question of if, but when.* Once again, I strengthen my resolve to turn all negative, frustrating experiences into positives, but that is the future, and this is now. It is time to put my words into actions.

I begin meditating, and as I am about to split my chi into two meridians on either side of my spine, while also directing my chi in the centerline meridian, the doubts kick in. A little mouthy New England attitude breaks through any uncertainty. Next, I apply the secret of success: practice, practice, practice. I am pleasantly surprised how simple it is to deepen my inner awareness and to split and guide my chi through three meridians. Surprisingly, there were very few locks to break through. In less than a month, it is second nature to guide and follow my chi comets in the three meridians, and it is a magnificent experience.

I thoroughly enjoy cleaning the three meridians which again

invigorates and helps my chi to flow freely. With each circulation, my inner awareness naturally deepens, and the three chi comets are even brighter, stronger, more invigorated, and faster. I am experiencing an even deeper level of peaceful, centered energy, and strength in and through my body; again, from the inside out. In addition, the gap between my inner world and the foreign outside world continues to narrow; I am almost in sync with the present time of the foreign outside world.

There are surprising and wonderful benefits. More and more, higher ranking Black Belts are asking me for help with their testing material, especially with their internal martial art forms. As I go through the forms and answer questions, I am treated with respect and as an equal. When we finish, most people thank me and continue to treat me well. However, there are a few people who, after they own their forms, try to reattach *their* label on me of a broken person who needs help and is incapable of helping others. I know their negative, unhealthy label is how they think and feel about themselves, it's not about me or anyone else. Compassionately, I look them squarely in the eye, even though they cannot look me in the eye, and politely ask if there's anything else I can help them with. They shift their weight side to side and their voices trail off as they say no. Maybe one day, they will decide to change directions; their mind-set and flow with life rather than against; it only takes a moment.

Winter has taken hold and instead of focusing on the cold and yuck, I concentrate on my next right step; circulating my chi out of my torso and into the limbs. Once again, the doubts start rearing their ugly heads. I know I can guide and follow my chi through three meridians, but how the heck am I going to circulate my chi through my arms and legs with a TBI? Will I be able to do it and how long will it take?

Immediately, my no B.S. attitude fires up. Frig the doubts – fear, stomp on it with both feet, and kick it to the curb. I remind myself how far I have come, and all the phenomenal things I have accomplished when no one else gave me any hope. I didn't know how to write a sentence, and a gnat had better focus and memory than I.

Next, I set my route. My inner awareness will deepen and be fine tuned by breaking through one lock and make one connection at a time as guide my chi through my entire body. Besides, I have a great foundation to build upon; I have already split and connected the three meridians in my upper body. Keep it simple, Cathy. *It's Easy* to circulate my chi into my arms and legs.

With my mind-set squared away, I step by step break through blockages and make connections; guiding, splitting, and following my chi as it circulates through the pathways in my torso, arms, and legs. As always, I practice simultaneously circulating my five chi comets until it becomes second nature. Once again, I am surprised how relatively easy and simple it is to simultaneously guide and follow all five vibrant chi comets. Next, I clean up the five pathways which invigorates and increases the chi's velocity.

It is very early spring 1999, and the pace of my brain healing journey continues to accelerate. *Each lock and meridian I have opened, connected, and cleaned has deepened my inner awareness to new and greater levels, and all five chi comets are stunningly bright, energetic, and quick.* I feel more like the real me, and I am thoroughly enjoying the enormous positive changes in all areas of my life. I am stronger, more energetic, balanced, centered, clearer, and beyond grateful. Now, it makes sense why I needed to move my chi out of my torso and into my extremities.

My next right step is to circulate the chi in a continuous wave through my body, rather than focus on an acupuncture point or meridians. With each continual wave of chi, I am aware of the magnificent flow of life giving chi. I am even more invigorated, balanced, peaceful, clear, present, and strong. I thought I knew what powerful, balanced energy was; I did not have a clue. I must be getting close to completely healing my brain.

25

BEING -
SPRING 1999

My next right step is to open and clean the main meridians in my body, one by one. With each meridian I open and clean, my brain healing journey accelerates to a whole new level. I have a gut sense to take a temporary break and work on enhancing my organs, a common meditation technique. Even though I do not believe in invigorating the organs, especially using different colors, I am open and will do my absolute best.

I locate each organ: heart, liver, lungs, kidneys, and spleen using anatomy drawings. Each organ has a specific color; heart – red, liver – green, lungs – white, kidneys – black, spleen – yellow. Although I don't have concrete proof that this color and invigoration thing works, it feels like I am getting an extra dose of energy. More importantly, my inner awareness continues to natural deepen and is now *precise*. Now, it is second nature to zoom in like a microscope revealing minute details of my inner being. There are no words to adequately describe my new level of precise inner awareness. As I have stated, again and again, my inner awareness training has to be experienced, and I will need to teach my method in person; otherwise, it is just intellectual information which is absolutely useless.

After I have enhanced my organs, I return to opening my meridians, one at a time. Months pass, and I am having a lot of fun. But, I am long past the point of needing to deepen my inner awareness training with this process; it is second nature to break through blockages, make connections, and open and clean meridians. A couple of months ago I was ready to move on; though, I do not know my next right step. I continue opening meridians, and since it is completely natural to do, it is very easy to focus on other things while meditating.

I ponder the term *body and mind*. Pre-TBI I thought of my body and mind as one, but I also felt there was a divide or a disconnection between my body and mind. It was so much easier to know and understand my body compared to what little I and others knew of the brain.

Before I began my brain healing journey, I had read and listened to people talk about the body and mind being one. Although they were speaking of them as one, I got a clear sense they were still making a distinction between the body and mind – brain. I believe this is not from a lack of intellectual information, but from not personally experiencing their brain and how it works from the inside, without machines, testing, etc.

I have a strong gut sense that I am on the road to connecting my body and mind into one by personally being aware and experiencing my brain from the inside. Although this is fascinating, it is just mental gymnastics. To know if my gut sense is right, I need to find a way to break through the prison in my brain, climb out of this never-ending hole, and be reconnected.

I continue to clear one meridian, and I am inwardly guided to the next. While meditating, I chuckle inside at how far I've come. I was just pondering "body and mind" and "being one." My inner awareness training is the gift that keeps on giving, and I trust that when it is the right time, the next right step will naturally emerge.

It's early autumn 1999, and I am opening the gall bladder

meridian, specifically GB 37 in my lower right leg when a scene from an old movie flashes across my mind. I do not know the name of the film, but considering what I am doing, the memory is rather intriguing. In the movie, the technology had been developed to shrink a submarine, including the people in it, small enough to go into the human body, explore, and heal the body. I continue to meditate, and wonder what is the significance of this memory and why is it happening now? Immediately I have a strong gut sense; it's time to go into the brain.

26

A SIMPLE DECISION IT'S EASY OR IT'S HARD?

I finish meditating and become aware of a profound weight in and on me. The pressure is coming from all the doubts and questions about me – the one with a TBI – entering the brain. Carefully, I listen to my thoughts and hear the very loud words of all the "no's and never-sayers." "We know very little about the brain" "The brain is too complex to understand." "We're in the infancy of understanding the brain." *I take a deep breath and take responsibility for my thinking and attitude, not theirs.* I am holding on to what the medical professionals and others have said and continue to say about the brain.

To change my perspective, I reflect on a time when I thought the body was too complex and would be too difficult to understand. Regardless, I kept persevering. Step by step, I delved deeper into my #1 brain healing technique: my inner awareness training and my results have been off the charts awesome, even by my standards. Should I study the medical models of the brain? How will they help? I already know the vast majority of damage is in my left temporal lobe and I know its location. I have been shown the plastic brain model with the removable lobes over and over and over again. The problem has been pounded into me; enough is enough. I need to keep seeking a solution. In my mind, I hear the simple and profound saying – if I keep positively thinking and speaking that a task will be easy and consistently take healthy actions – most likely it will be easier – no matter how many people say it's impossible or difficult to do.

Again, I set my sights higher than anyone else thinks is possible because that is where everything is possible. I am 100% committed to discovering a solution to the TBI – it is irrelevant that there isn't a guide, a book, or a pamphlet to show me how to completely heal and enhance my brain better than before. I will discover a solution.

Next, I make a conscious decision not to talk with my friends or anyone else about my decision to enter the brain and the discoveries I will make. I will wait until after I have made significant progress then I will share my discoveries. I do not want even a hint of doubt from anyone. Again, my quiet determination mode kicks in. Keep it simple. *It's Easy* to completely heal and enhance my brain better than before the TBI!

PHASE 3

A NEW ERA

COMPLETELY
HEALING
AND
ENHANCING
MY BRAIN

27

AN EXPLORATION INTO UNCHARTED TERRITORY EARLY AUTUMN 1999

With a new perspective, I look at my brain as just another organ which needs to be invigorated, balanced, completely healed, and enhanced. I do not have any expectations of how the process will unfold. I do have complete trust. I will liberate myself and be reconnected.

I begin meditating and when I am calmly aware and connected, I innately switch my attention to the right side of my head. Once again, I clean up the meridians. The gall bladder meridian in particular is an absolute delight to guide my chi through; the zigs, zags, and sweeping movements of my chi as it effortlessly flows around my right ear is better than any amusement ride.

Next, my inner awareness shifts to invigorating my brain organ. I have a gut sense to rejuvenate and balance the right hemisphere of my brain, just as I did with my chi, meridians, and organs. Every day for weeks I do my training, and with each meditation, my right hemisphere feels healthier and a little more balanced. There is even a bit of lightness in my right hemisphere, not in weight, but in brightness which is very encouraging considering it was totally black.

In the middle of a meditation, I notice a very small blip of light. No, it's more of a starburst. I begin to focus on the area where the light originated when another starburst lights up a very short distance away. This is remarkable. Though, I have no idea what just happened.

Incrementally, I deepen my inner awareness by slowing the pace of my meditation. I am aware of more and more starbursts though it's difficult to follow and make out their details. Again, I intentionally deepen my inner awareness. The process of deepening my inner awareness reminds me of how my eyes slowly adjust when I enter a dark room; this helps me to be more patient.

Rather quickly, I see each tiny starburst has a very dim trailing light. This minuscule comet in my brain is similar to the chi comet I first experienced between my tan tien and ming men, and then in every meridian. However, the starbursts with their trailing lights in my brain are microscopic compared to the ones in my meridians. I wonder. Could these starbursts be the key to unlocking the prison in my brain? Intentionally, I deepen my inner awareness, and my mini light show becomes immense and much too quick to follow.

My next meditation, I purposefully slow the pace of my meditation to be more in sync with the starbursts and their energetic movements. I am intrigued by the efficiency, speed, and precision of the starbursts and the minute space between each starburst; it is beautiful and most impressive. After much observation and deliberation, I come up with a theory. Each starburst and connecting starburst is a thought or a function my brain is performing in another part of my body.

The next meditation, I naturally deepen my inner awareness. My right hemisphere becomes luminous with an immeasurable amount of starbursts. I feel like I have been invited into the most majestic secret room and it's – inside me! I sense I am in sync with the energy of the starbursts in my brain. Next, I see a sight which I haven't seen in years **DAYLIGHT!** *Far above me in the never-ending hole is a radiant light! Although I am not able to see the opening, I must be getting closer to liberating and reconnecting myself. In each step of my brain healing journey, I have trusted and believed I was climbing in the right direction, but I didn't know for certain – until now. I am in awe and profoundly grateful. My beacon of hope is coming from inside my brain. What a magnificent view!*

My next meditation, I move to just inside my right temporal lobe and consciously deepen my inner awareness. I concentrate on having a thought – a starburst lights up – my thought finishes and another starburst lights up. I am stunned and ecstatic! I have just experienced the connecting of two synapses! I start to lose my inner awareness and quickly center myself.

Rather than move forward, I decide to take stock while meditating. I have discovered a way to enter my brain, and have developed the ability to invigorate my brain. I know how to intentionally and incrementally deepen my inner awareness to be in sync with my brain. I have also discovered how a thought originates and is completed when it connects with or lights up another starburst or synapse. I am experiencing a new era of brain exploration, or maybe a more precise term is – lighting up a new era in brain exploration.

With each meditation I become more impressed with the light show which continues to emerge in my right hemisphere and right temporal lobe. While observing the vast quantity of luminous starbursts, light tails, and connections, I have another Ah ha, knock my socks off moment. My perspective of how I perceive myself has changed. There is no longer a separation of mind and body. I am one whole being! From this point forward, I will not differentiate between my body and mind; I am one and will describe myself as – being or one being.

Methodically, I continue until it becomes difficult to follow the vast array of lights and connections in my right temporal lobe. I deepen my meditation to be aware of a single star burst, how it travels, and the connection. For the first time, I am aware and connected to a pathway. I follow and study numerous pathways in my brain which are different than the meridian system. The pathways in my brain are more of a very thin wire, whereas the meridians are thicker, wider, and hollow or tubular in shape.

As I'm about to end a meditation, I have a gut sense that it's time to switch my focus to my left hemisphere. At first, I am a little surprised, until I realize my inner awareness training in my right hemisphere and right temporal lobe has become second nature which means it's time for my next right step.

Before moving forward I decide to take stock. For the first time since the accident, the thick, blurry glass prison in my brain is a little thinner and not as blurry! Also, the light at the top of the never-ending hole is brighter and wider! Although I am still not able to see the opening, I must be getting closer. My thinking is quicker and clearer, and more importantly, I have incrementally deepened my inner awareness, step by step. Inwardly I celebrate; I am thankful I have kept my decision about going into my brain and discoveries to myself. If I had shared my world-changing discoveries right after I experienced them, I am not sure if people's reactions would have taken me off-course. Again, this is something I am not willing to risk. I decide to take time to enjoy and contemplate my monumental news before sharing it.

Later, I enthusiastically share all my earth-shaking news with my friends, including the phenomenal changes in the thick, blurry glass wall, and how it feels like I am home in my right hemisphere and right temporal lobe. Next, I share my hesitancy to enter the left hemisphere. I conclude with a theory. With this giant leap forward, I believe I am very close to liberating myself from the prison in my brain.

SILENCE. In time, I will get used to the 10 – 15 seconds of stunned looks and hush that comes over the room when I explain my method and ground-breaking discoveries, but for now, it is rather perplexing. If the situation were reversed, I would be asking questions and for more details, and explanations about the brain and the brain healing training. People tell me they do not know what to say. They see and have seen all of my steady improvements and huge accomplishments at each step of my brain healing journey. But, they do not know what to say when it comes to my stunning brain discoveries. After a few minutes their responses change; here is one that describes people's sentiment. "Cathy, what you have discovered and all the advancements you have made are world-changing! You need to keep going and move into the left hemisphere of your brain! Cathy, you also need to write a book, you could help so many people!"

My answer to writing a book is always the same – it is the last thing I want to do. For years, people have asked me to write a book about my life. But, I would rather be digging ditches in the middle of winter, in the rocky soil of New England during a Nor'easter, than write a book about myself. What I do not tell them is it would take thousands and thousands of pages to explain everything I have done so far, but it would still be incomplete, because my method needs to be taught in person.

I shift the conversation towards the brain, my discoveries, how I delved deeper into my inner awareness training and my brain healing journey, but that is the last thing people want to talk about. I do not understand. Are people stuck on the concept that it is "impossible" to heal the brain, and the brain is too complex to understand? I do not know. Though, I am grateful I have not believed, bought into, and fed the negativity of other people's "no's and never's" and "impossibles," especially when it comes to the brain. In every cell of my being, I know It's Easy to completely heal my brain. I am steps away.

28

CREATING MY
FIRST SYNAPSE
CONNECTION

I set my sights on entering my left hemisphere. I am calm, hopeful, a little excited, and unsure. I begin meditating and when I am calmly aware and connected in my right hemisphere, I easily move into my left hemisphere. I am stunned! The bleakness of this decrepit, dark, sort of gray, lifeless gooey texture is disheartening to say the least. My first reaction is to rush back to my vibrant right hemisphere which is bathed in brilliant light and filled with lightning-quick, purposeful connections.

I look at my left temporal lobe. I am utterly shocked. There are no signs of life; it is completely dark. I notice disjointed, mangled connections between my left temporal lobe and the adjoining lobes. They are a total contrast to the smooth, seamless, energetic connections between the lobes in my right hemisphere. I take a deep breath and slowly exhale which keeps me calm, aware, and connected while meditating. The massive contrast between the two hemispheres is another great incentive to completely heal my brain.

I begin invigorating and balancing the dark gray gooey texture which makes up my left hemisphere, just as I have done with my chi, meridians, organs, and right hemisphere. In particular, I am working on a rather large area between the mid-line of my brain and the area outside my left temporal lobe. While meditating, a memory flashes across my mind of when I hurt my right knee years before the TBI. The orthopedic doctor suggested that my healthy knee would help teach my damaged knee how to heal. Now, I understand my gut sense to begin my brain exploration in my intact, healthy right hemisphere. I needed to further develop my inner awareness to experience how the healthy side of my brain works and makes connections (right hemisphere and right temporal lobe) in order to take another step towards completely healing my brain.

I take an extra long time invigorating and balancing my left hemisphere – more than is necessary – two weeks. Next, I become intrigued with the gray, gooey lifeless texture and decide to find out what is working. Purposefully, I have a thought. To my amazement, a barely visible miniscule starburst lights up nearby. The starburst with its trailing light begins to move very lethargically. Quickly, I map where the starburst originated with an X, Y, and Z and call it synapse "A". In time, I will name this tool my Internal Brain Mapping Technique. I follow the starburst as I have followed every chi comet from my tan tien to ming men, in every meridian, in my right hemisphere, and right temporal lobe. Though this pathway is vastly different; it is curved, and again, the starburst is extremely sluggish; this is a complete contrast to the rather straight, lightening-quick, precise, and extremely short pathways in my right hemisphere. The starburst has been traveling in my left hemisphere for a very long time, both in distance about four inches, and length of time, when another miniscule, dim starburst lights up as my thought is completed. I am astounded by the length of time and space that it took to complete a single thought, and I am extraordinarily thankful. For the first time since the TBI, I fully understand why it takes so long to complete a single thought in my left hemisphere. Before

I end my meditation, I map the second starburst connection as synapse "B" with an X, Y, and Z.

Again, I contemplate my world-changing discoveries before sharing them with my friends. Once more, they are stunned for 10 – 15 seconds; then, they encourage me to keep persevering. The consensus is to shorten the distance between the two synapses, but no one knows how to close the gap. I walk away thinking; how the heck am I going to close the distance between these two synapses?

I sit down to my next meditation without any idea of how to close the gap, though I have complete trust. I will develop a solution. When I am calmly aware and connected in my left hemisphere, I easily move to synapse "A" which is where my thought originated from my previous meditation. There has to be a way to make a more precise, direct pathway between synapses "A" and "B." Maybe, it's similar to how my right hemisphere works. Consciously, I decide to shorten the distance between the two synapses. Once again, I embark at synapse "A" by purposely having a thought. Thankfully, it is second nature to follow starbursts in my brain, which makes it easy to switch the majority of my inner awareness to how to close the gap between the two synapses.

A thought crosses my mind. How would I land a plane? As I am approaching synapse "B," I intensify my inner awareness by looking for my new destination: the synapse directly in front of synapse "B." Immediately, I see my new synapse connection "C." Intentionally I deepen my meditation, but the pace of the miniscule starburst remains the same. With every ounce of inner awareness I can muster, I calmly place all my focus on connecting with synapse "C." Immediately, I feel a slight vacuum effect drawing the starburst into the new synapse. The vacuum effect reminds me of rooting, especially when I do my internal martial art forms. In an instant, the starburst connects with synapse "C!" The ease of making a new synapse connection is impressive!

While trying to comprehend the significance of another mammoth earth-shattering achievement and discovery, my brain automatically picks up the task of systematically making new synapse connections between "A" and "C" – always starting at synapse "A!" In awe, I am aware and watching my brain playing another version of ping pong regeneration. With each new synapse connection, the pathway becomes straighter, and the starburst and light tail becomes brighter, more vigorous, and faster! Simultaneously, my thinking and world becomes clearer and a little brighter! An almost straight line of synapses is being reconnected! This is magnificent, I had no idea my brain could automatically close the gap! Once again, I get the sense my brain has been waiting for me to do my task of, step by step, delving deeper into my inner awareness training; in order for my brain to automatically begin the process of healing and reconnecting this pathway of synapses! While the automatic regeneration process continues, I map synapse "C" with an X, Y, and Z. I begin to map the next few synapses; "D" "E" and "F" but stop. Instead of mapping all the new synapses, I decide to enjoy this spectacular process. If I need to map the new connections, I will do it another time.

While meditating, I decide to take stock. The prison wall in my brain is even thinner and clearer, and the light above me in the never-ending hole is brilliant and wider! I marvel at the gorgeous opening, or what I believe is the opening because I am still not able to see it. How am I going to physically pull myself up and out of this hole? I know I am stronger, but am I that strong? Quickly, I square away my thinking. Cathy, first you have to get to the top, then you will figure it out. I change my perspective by deciding to thoroughly enjoy my new level of rejuvenation and clarity! It is impressive how simple, precise, and easy it is being aware and experiencing the new connections, and understanding my brain from the inside. Bottom line, the brain is not complicated or difficult to understand; it is just like the rest of my being. My brain wants and needs to be healthy, balanced, free, and reconnected.

I end my meditation and take time to ponder my world-changing discoveries. When I share my findings with my friends, they lean in as I explain that, while en route, the idea came to me to close the gap like I was landing an airplane. I finish speaking, and again, there is the 10 – 15 seconds of silence. Then, we talk about the significance of my discoveries, and how the next step is to find the lock on my left temporal lobe. Once again, no one knows how to locate the lock. I am on my own. How do I discover a way into my left temporal lobe?

29

FINDING THE LOCK

Before I meditate, I theorize about the location of the lock. The lock must be at the site of the original damage, where my brain bounced off the skull. Next, I become aware of my thinking. My most pressing thought is that although I am confident that I will find the lock, I am also a little saddened by the utter darkness and the immense damage of my left temporal lobe. Rather than feed the negative, I decide to square away my mind-set. As soon as I find the lock, I will be one step closer to liberating and reconnecting myself.

I begin meditating and when I am calmly and profoundly aware and connected in my left hemisphere, I consciously switch my attention and scan the outer layer of my left temporal lobe. I am using the same technique that I have utilized from day one of my brain healing journey – my inner awareness training. My search quickly reveals two injury sites on the outer layer of my left temporal lobe. Easily, I map each area with an X, Y, and Z using my Internal Brain Mapping Technique. I believe the first trauma occurred where my brain struck the skull, and the second trauma, which has less damage, was caused by the reverberation effect. Knowing the position of these two injury sites is great information, but the lock is not located at these damaged areas. My solution resides elsewhere.

Continuing my search, I figure it will take days, if not weeks, to locate the lock on the outer layer of my left temporal lobe. However, in a matter of minutes, I find the biggest lock I have ever faced and it looks – permanently bolted shut. I focus on how quickly I found the lock, where it's located, and why the lock is here and not at the two damaged areas. Ahh, I have switched my focus. If I keep looking at the where's, why's, and other questions, it will be a colossal waste of time and effort which will take me off-course. Before I can break through this mammoth lock, I need to be completely aware and connected. I finish my meditation in order to center myself and to get any and all distracting thoughts out of the way.

REFLECTION AND A THEORY

Looking in the mirror, I wonder what I will look like when I completely heal my brain. Will I look like I did before the TBI, only 10 years older? Will I be more vibrant? I do not know. Though, I do have a theory of how my left temporal lobe will begin to heal. I believe it will take days, or even weeks, to delve deep enough into my inner awareness training to generate enough chi to create even a miniscule crack in this massive lock. I theorize that the healing process will begin in the core of my left temporal lobe and incrementally work its way outward.

30

RE-BOOTING MY
LEFT TEMPORAL
LOBE
AUTUMN 1999

I have a gut sense that I am on the verge of a massive discovery, one of the biggest ever. I am also intimidated by the immensity of this lock and the lifelessness of my left temporal lobe. Again, I square away my mind-set by reminding myself that, step by step, I have developed and fine tuned my inner awareness and brain healing training, and I have broken through all kinds of locks. *I am ready to break through this lock, make the connection, liberate, and reconnect myself. Before I begin meditating, I say to my self; It's Easy to completely heal my brain.*

I take a deep breath, center myself, slowly exhale, and begin meditating. When I am calmly and profoundly aware and connected, I easily move to the massive lock on my left temporal lobe. Step by step, I incrementally deepen my inner awareness, but each and every attempt to break through the lock is unsuccessful. I need to delve deeper into my inner awareness training. I end my meditation and contemplate my next right move.

Later, I share my quandary with my friends. I am asked to think of the biggest tool a person can hold. The first thought that crosses my mind is a jack hammer. Immediately, I think of the strongest person in the world using a jackhammer to break through the lock on my left temporal lobe. My friends encourage me to keep persevering, but once again, no one knows how to help me.

Before my next meditation, I make a couple of decisions. First, I will upgrade my chi pointed woodworking tool to a chi jackhammer and will visualize the strongest person in the world using the chi jackhammer to bust through the lock. My second decision squares away my mind-set. I will tenaciously focus on breaking through this lock as if my life depends on it.

I begin my second meditation and when I am calmly and profoundly aware and connected, I switch my attention to surveying the topography of this immense lock. In some areas the lock is relatively smooth, where others it is quite rough. In many ways the lock looks like a thick scar or scab, the kind that are on knees and elbows. I decide to find the deepest, thinnest, and weakest area which hopefully will be the easiest area to break through. This certainly makes more sense than the strategy of trying to break through the entirety of this mammoth lock.

Continuing my scan, I notice an area which is quite rugged compared to the rest. Within this region is a particular large peak, and right next to it is the deepest valley of the entire lock. I believe the valley will be the best location to break through the lock. Purposefully, I deepen my meditation by intensely focusing on the deepest part of the valley. I fine tune my inner awareness to a very precise area. After a few minutes a small crack appears. Consciously, I stop using the visualization of the chi jackhammer and strong person. Intentionally I deepen my inner awareness into the breach, and instantaneously, the lock bursts wide open without any pain! My left temporal lobe lights up like fireworks on a 4th of July night! The outermost layer is automatically flickering on *similar to an older version of a fluorescent light bulb! Layer by layer, the illuminating, pulsating energy is working its way inward! This is one of the most spectacular experiences and sights of my entire life! There are no words in any language that can fully express this phenomenal, luminous light; it has to be experienced!*

Next, my left temporal lobe automatically begins to re-boot while the lighting up process continues to move inward, layer by layer! As my left temporal lobe is awakening, my thought process is improving; at the same rate! Being aware of and experiencing connections and watching this extraordinary, simultaneous regeneration is electric, literally! The automatic re-booting process of my left temporal lobe is similar to how my brain automatically reconnected the synapses in my left hemisphere, but there are differences. The automatic re-booting of my left temporal lobe is more of a global or whole event encompassing a vast array of functions and reconnections. Whereas, the automatic synapse reconnecting process in my left hemisphere was more of a singular function.

The automatic re-booting of my left temporal lobe continues. Much of this immense process I am not able to follow, but that doesn't matter because I am thoroughly enjoying the quantity, quality, and speed with which I can think, remember, and retrieve information! It is effortless! There is no work to think; it just is!

My left temporal lobe is now two thirds re-booted, and I experience a tremendous awakening and fullness within my brain, especially in my left temporal lobe, that I didn't know was missing! In order to be balanced, I have to physically compensate my meditation posture. After I re-center, a small flickering ripple in my left temporal lobe changes into a larger automatic re-boot wave – my second – which begins to reconnect my left temporal lobe with the adjacent lobes! However, the automatic reconnecting process of my left temporal lobe with the bordering lobes is quite different than the seamless connections between the lobes in my right hemisphere.

Emerging from my left temporal lobe are individual *connections attaching and reconnecting only to the outer layer of each adjoining lobe. More precisely, each single reconnection is occurring at very precise locations with large spaces between them. The second individual* reconnections are occurring right alongside each original connection. The third, fourth, etc., individual reconnections are forming into round clusters. When the reconnections reach their maximum capacity point, these major reconnections penetrates deep into the bordering lobes. Instantly, other reconnections from my left temporal lobe fill in the spaces between each major reconnection, and they are attaching into the adjoining lobes. Wow, I am coming home!

I have a gut sense that each major reconnection from my left temporal lobe are the main, most crucial functions that had to be reattached first. I sense the bordering lobes were making sure these main reconnections were viable, healthy, and had enough power before they were accepted and allowed to enter the lobes. From there, all the other reconnections were able to connect next to these powerful, healthy main pathways. The main reconnections remind me of when a bone is broken and is completely healed, the area is much stronger. The main reconnections from my left temporal lobe to the adjoining lobes are larger and much stronger than the connections in my right hemisphere.

The automatic re-booting of my left temporal lobe concludes. As my left temporal lobe continues to be reattached to the adjacent lobes, I am pleasantly surprised how precise my thinking has become. It's taken one minute twenty seven seconds to one minute twenty eight seconds to re-boot my left temporal lobe. Wow, why does my brain like; no – need to be so extremely precise? Quickly I ponder the question and realize my brain or thinking being precise is my natural or normal state of being. Was my brain that precise pre- TBI? I do not know. I believe that, before the TBI, I was not aware and connected enough to notice. Should I focus on the length of time of each automatic re-boot and why my thinking is so precise? Consciously, I decide to thoroughly enjoy this magnificent experience. My brain is healing!

With my mind-set squared away – my third automatic re-boot wave begins reconnecting my left temporal lobe to my entire brain, while my left temporal lobe continues to be reunited with its adjoining lobes! Being aware, experiencing, and watching this impressive healing and reintegrating process leads me to another enormous insight! The solution to completely heal my brain has been inside me the entire time I had the TBI! From the moment the injury occurred, my brain has been *waiting for me to do my job to – step by step, delve deeper into my inner awareness and brain healing training, in order to develop my method, before my brain could begin to do its job.*

My entire brain has finished re-booting, and I experience a slightly larger automatic re-boot wave – my fourth which is reintegrating my entire anatomy from head to toe! A radiant light has been switched on illuminating my whole being from the inside out! I am filled with a profound sense of peace, clarity, centeredness, gratitude, and love! For the first time since the TBI, I am no longer disconnected. I am a whole being. I am one and full of life!

The automatic re-booting and reintegrating processes seems to have subsided. I am not sure if what I am experiencing is a lull, or if my brain has completed the healing process. In a state of bliss, I continue patiently meditating.

During the automatic re-booting and reintegrating process, I had many gut senses happening almost simultaneously, and decided not to give them my full attention, until now. Here are a few. I realize that I did not have a busted brain or brain damage, I had – disconnections in my brain. To break through the lock and make these reconnections, my job was to, step by step, develop my whole method. The brain has a tremendous need to completely heal itself.

In addition, I need to precisely teach people throughout the world; people with intact brains and people with disconnections in the brain how to completely heal the brain. I am most interested in teaching people to become instructors; people with intact brains and with disconnections in the brain; then, they can return to their state or country and using the same high standard teach others. What an amazing concept – people who were imprisoned in their brain will liberate themselves; then, teach others how to completely heal the brain! I am really looking forward to meeting positive transformation warriors. (At the time, I was open to teach anyone; however, later in the book I will clarify the required qualifications to be a student, a staff member, and the organizations who work for and with me.)

Next, in what other ways will my whole method help others, and how can I improve my method? My focus shifts. How am I going to reach people throughout the world? I am just one person. A few seconds later, I decide to trust; my answers will come.

When I am absolutely sure the process of completely healing and reintegrating my brain is complete, I end my meditation and inwardly celebrate! I have completely healed my brain from the TBI! The moment I broke through the lock on and in my left temporal lobe and made the connection, the thick, blurry prison wall ceased to exist! The impossible is now possible! I feel like a phoenix rising from the ashes – a Brain Phoenix ™. What once seemed inconceivable has now become a reality! I have kept my promise and liberated myself! At will, I am using my brain again, and all at once, I want to think, speak, remember, move, reconnect with people, and fully live my life! I love how easy it is to think and remember. I love the balanced powerhouse of vivacious energy and strength that is invigorating me from the inside out! I have completely healed my brain, and I will not take my ability to think and use my brain for granted, ever again!

I look in the mirror and absolutely love the view! There are no signs of TBI in my eyes or on my face! I see the real me: an intelligent, athletic, friendly, energetic human being full of joy! The depth of gratitude is immeasurable; every cell in my being is bursting with gratitude! My brain is completely healed, reconnected, and I am a whole being!

I let out a huge belly laugh – it has taken a person with a busted brain; no with – disconnections in the brain – to figure out how to completely heal the brain from the inside! Now, I understand that a person, who had disconnections in their brain, and who was absolutely committed to finding a solution was the only person who could develop an inner solution – my inner awareness training and my whole method – Brain Phoenix ™. I needed to do my job, and do it thoroughly, in order for my brain to do its job! I also believe I had the exact amount of disconnections in my brain to develop this inner solution. If I had had more disconnections, I might not have been able to develop my method. On the other hand, if I had had a lot less disconnections in my brain, I might not have had such a strong desire to keep persevering and I might have settled for less. Ahh, the heck with all the "what ifs and what might have beens" that is a colossal waste of time and energy! I am going to thoroughly enjoying the gift of the present moment and the magnitude of this world-changing event! I am free and giddy with gratitude! There are no words to adequately express what it is like to liberate myself. To fully comprehend this exquisite freedom, a person has to experience it.

Reflecting upon my whole brain healing journey, I calculate that it has taken a little less than three years to emancipate myself – not counting the time for the initial trauma to subside, the missteps, and the dead-end paths. Heck, I'm even thankful for the missteps and the ten years plus to blaze this trail! My inner celebration continues, and I realize where I am at with the never-ending hole.

31

A QUESTION OF RECONNECTING

In my mind's eye, I lift my right knee out of the never-ending hole. For the first time, I kneel on solid ground and give thanks for completely healing my brain, for my freedom, and for my life! I stand up, dust myself off, and survey my surroundings. I am alone in a semi-desert environment. There are small bushes interspersed as far as the eye can see. Off in the distance is a medium-size mountain range which looks rather lush compared to my surroundings. I surmise if I am going to find people, the best place is over there by those green mountains.

Before I can move, I need to make a conscious decision. Do I want to reconnect with Divine Source, the people I love, and the world? WHAT! Why do I have to make a conscious decision to reconnect? Of course, I want to be reconnected! Why isn't reconnecting a part of the automatic brain rebooting and reintegrating process? I am stunned, and a little ticked off, not only for myself, but what about other people? Will other people with disconnections in their brain from an accident or disease have to make this decision after I have taught them my whole Brain Phoenix ™ method? Will people who have been locked inside their brains their entire lives have to choose? Will they know the difference between their inner brain world and the foreign outside world? Will they decide to stay in their brain? I do not know.

Arrghh, I do not understand why I *have* to make this decision. Why isn't being reconnected a part of completely healing my brain? *Everything* I did was to free myself in order to be reconnected! Wasn't it bad enough to be imprisoned in my brain? I am surprised more people don't go mad being isolated within their brain. WHY do I have to make a decision to be reconnected?

Regardless of how frustrating this is, I am not able to move forward until I make a conscious decision to reconnect. Though I do not understand, I am extremely grateful to have a choice. YES, I want to be reconnected! Of course, I want to be reconnected! Immediately, I'm able to begin my journey towards the lush green mountains.

I take another 360 degree panoramic view, and see something which catches my eye. The never-ending hole behind me no longer exists; it has been filled in and looks like the rest of the area. I am not exactly sure what this means, but I decide to take it as a sign of encouragement. Rather than focusing on where I came from and why I had to make a conscious decision to be reconnected. I exuberantly begin the next part of my journey. Smiling from ear to ear, I walk towards the lush green mountains!

A UNIQUE
CELEBRATION

For years, I have dreamt about how I would celebrate completely healing my brain, liberating myself, and being reconnected. I saw myself in pure ecstasy, jumping up and down with my arms overhead shouting as loud as I could. I COMPLETELY HEALED MY BRAIN! I AM FREE! I HAVE EMANCIPATED MYSELF! THE THICK, BLURRY GLASS PRISON IN MY BRAIN NO LONGER EXISTS! I CAN THINK AGAIN! I CAN REMEMBER AGAIN! AT WILL, I AM USING MY BRAIN! I AM FREE!!!

My celebration is very different – again, it is mostly on the inside. Maybe it's because I still have to be reconnected with people. Could it be that I freed myself and celebrating my independence is something I want to keep to myself? No, that's not it; even though, there is a small part of me that wants to keep what happened to my self. Is it because I spent so many years disconnected and imprisoned in my brain?

I take time to ponder these and other questions. I come to the conclusion that I do not know and may never know the answers. I also put my unusual celebration into perspective – it does not matter. I have completely healed my brain, and now, I am heading towards being reconnected with people! Life is good!

32

STUNNING
DEVELOPMENTS

My interactions with people are deepening, and I have had many remarkable experiences. Here are a few. In numerous conversations with different people, I find myself finishing a sentence and perplexingly asking myself out loud, "How do I know the word ____, (fill in the blank) and how do I know the definition?" I know that I am using the words correctly, but I do not think I knew these words pre-TBI.

After much reflection, I come to the conclusion that, during the automatic re-booting and reintegrating process, connections were made to information that was already in my brain. Once again, rather than focusing on the why's and how come's, I decide to thoroughly enjoy the boost in my vocabulary.

Second, my brain still needs to be extremely precise, especially with numbers, which first occurred during the automatic re-booting process. Instead of saying that a project is 85% complete. I now say, "The project is 84.628 complete, more precisely it is between 84.628 to 85.225 complete." Usually people laugh and ask if I can be more specific. Though, I still do not totally understand why my brain needs to be so precise. In time, I will make peace with the precision, and before speaking, I will take a moment to standardize my response even though my brain continually insists on being extremely precise.

Third, although my memory is not perfect, I now remember events which occurred during the period that I had the TBI. When I talk with friends and family to verify, my memories are always spot on. This experience completely changes my previous beliefs about memory, especially short term memory. I now believe all memories, words etc. get into the brain, and it is a matter of connecting to and retrieving them.

Fourth, my ability as a teacher of a martial art continues to improve. Once again, I introduce my brain healing techniques including my inner awareness to students; though, I call them techniques that have helped me. At first, I am met with resistance. I change my approach. Here is one example. I ask a student, "What are you working on, and what are your goals?" After we have trained for a bit, and if it is appropriate, I ask what they do and what they love to do. Or as I like to say, "What makes your heart sing?" Usually, somewhere in the conversation, their energy changes, their eyes light up, and their body becomes animated as they talk about what they love to do.

Instinctively, I switch how I explain the martial art techniques, movements, forms, and information in the language that makes their heart sing, whether it is mechanical, biology, artistic, etc. To be clear, we are all speaking English. By adapting my words, and how I explain inner awareness and other techniques, it makes it easier and quicker for people to understand, apply, and own the movements and forms. When I explain how I am teaching, some people tell me they are a visual or a verbal learner. I explain that how I teach is a simultaneous approach, not a singular approach. By utilizing my techniques simultaneously, it is easier to own information and forms. Even though I get a few strange looks, most people appreciate owning their forms a little quicker, and the thorough, simple manner in which I teach. I am grateful that it is completely natural to utilize what I have experienced and learned in my brain healing journey to teach people from all different backgrounds, education and martial art levels.

Although there are many positive developments from completely healing my brain, there is one snag. I am having difficulty speaking some multi-syllable words that I have not spoken since the accident. It's like I have a stutter, but I absolutely know that is not the problem. I do not understand why the automatic process of re-booting and reintegrating my brain did not fix this glitch. Again, focusing on the why's and how come's will not get the job done. Instead, I practice each multi-syllable word in my mind, then out loud, over and over again. Unfortunately, my progress is very slow and incomplete. Rather quickly, I come to the conclusion that I am using an outer method to fix an inner problem. I need to delve deeper into my inner awareness training to discover another inner solution.

33

ENHANCING MY BRAIN RECONNECTING MY LIFE AND A LIFETIME OF BRAIN EXPLORATION AND EDUCATION

My brain exploration continues. I need to be better than before the TBI. I begin meditating, and when I am calmly aware and connected, I easily enter my healthy, vibrant brain; then, effortlessly move into my very lively left temporal lobe. Quickly, I discover that I am having difficulty locating words in my left temporal lobe. I also do not know where the challenge is occurring with my mouth. I speak a few multi-syllable words while naturally deepening my inner awareness which quickly solves the mystery. The precise location of the blockage is with my lips; they have forgotten how to mold themselves around some multi-syllable words. I am absolutely shocked how easy and quick it is to diagnose the problem and the specific location. The challenge isn't with my vocal cords, tongue, or the rest of my mouth; it is with my lips. I take a moment to enjoy another world-changing discovery. I love my precious inner awareness training.

I modify my meditation to meditating in daily life, as I did shortly after my 3 Day Inner Awareness Training to the Tan Tien. The reason for the change in how I meditate is the necessity of; (1) Speaking each word out loud in order to locate the words *in* my left temporal lobe. (2) To discover a solution to reconnect my lips and anything else that needs to be reconnected in order to easily speak. Next, I make the most of my mind-set *It's Easy* to focus on my next right step. Out loud I say, "Creating a connection to my lips, and discovering where words are located in my left temporal lobe is a good challenge, and it will be simple and easy to eloquently speak again."

I begin by speaking a multi-syllable word out loud. Instantaneously, a vibrant starburst lights up *in* my left temporal lobe, which I precisely map with an X, Y, and Z using my Internal Brain Mapping Technique. To my surprise and delight, even when I'm having trouble speaking a word, the exact area lights up. Again, I speak each multi-syllable word numerous times, making sure I have correctly marked the location *in* my left temporal lobe in order to quickly retrieve the words in the future.

Next, I am aware of the physical location of my lips *on* my face, and how to move my lips while speaking each word. Diligently, I practice each word and phrase out loud, and my speech improves by leaps and bounds. Although my rate of improvement is extraordinarily fast, compared to the old, outer method, I wrestle with impatience. Fortunately, my resolve to continue improving at a steady rate wins over my immaturity. I finish my brain exploration work for the day. No, this isn't work. My brain exploration is so much fun, its play!

When I come across a multi-syllable word that I have not spoken since the accident, I have to go through the entire process of finding the word *in* my left temporal lobe, focusing on how to move my lips *on* my face while speaking the word over and over again. There has to be a better, simpler, and easier way to improve this process.

Quickly, I review each step and I have a monumental insight. In order to reconnect my words, lips, and speech, I need to simultaneously be aware of the location of a word *in* my left temporal lobe, the location of my lips *in* my brain, and the physical movements of my lips *on* my face; then, I need to simultaneously connect these three areas. I love it – another massive discovery!

To find my lips *in* my brain, I move my lips up and down without speaking which leads to an unusual and significant discovery. Thinking of a word and having emotion about that word, while moving my lips, creates a haze on the borders and slightly expands the boundaries where the lips are located *in* my brain. Intentionally, I deepen my inner awareness and move *my lips on my face without emotion*. Immediately, I am aware and see the precise area of *my lips in my brain lighting up*. As always, I repeat the process numerous times to confirm that I have the correct location. I use my Internal Brain Mapping Technique to easily map the location of my lips *in* my brain.

It's time to simultaneously connect the three areas. First, I locate a word *in* my left temporal lobe; then, the area where my lips are located *in* my brain, and finally, my lips *on* my face. My inner awareness naturally deepens as I simultaneously become aware of all three locations. Next, I slowly speak the multi-syllable word out loud allowing my lips to form around the word as it flows out my mouth. I practice being aware of all three locations until I am skillfully speaking the word. I choose another word and follow the same process. As I am choosing my third multi-syllable word, my brain automatically makes each separate connection into one connection (the location of a word *in* my left temporal lobe, the area where my lips are located *in* my brain, and my lips *on* my face) which speeds up and improves my speech. Next, I ingrain my method which naturally deepens my inner awareness, improves my brain function, and invigorates my whole being! My rate of verbal improvement is astonishingly fast! In time, I will name my process *Internal Brain Verbal and Physical Reconnecting Method.*

Months later, I face another interesting dilemma when I come across a multi-syllable word that I have not spoken since the accident. While I am utilizing my Internal Brain Verbal and Physical Reconnecting Method, I realize there has to be a better way to enhance my brain.

I decide to break everything down by *being aware of one connection at a time.* First, I focus on the location of a word *in* my left temporal lobe which, of course, lights up. Next, I follow the lighted pathway through the lobes in my brain until the connection is made with my lips *in* my brain. I am shocked; the connection in my brain is not direct. The pathway reminds me of an inefficient highway. At times, the pathway meanders, makes unusual sharp turns, and it is not level.

My first thought is to clean up the pathway. Immediately, I have a gut sense that I need to create a more precise route within my brain. Next, I turn my attention to how I closed the gap between synapses "A" and "B" in my left hemisphere and decide to improve on the technique.

I begin in my left temporal lobe and simultaneously become aware of all three locations: a word *in* my left temporal lobe, my lips *in* my brain, and my lips *on* my face. Next, I innately switch and deepen my inner awareness to the location of the word in my left temporal lobe *with the intent of creating a more direct route to my lips in my brain.*

Automatically, my brain re-routes a pathway by making a sort of a wide-ish, unusual turn then slowly reconnects a slightly more direct route to the lip area in my brain. As fast as lightning, the word fires to my mouth and easily flows out. Being aware and experiencing the connections, and watching my brain automatically make a new global pathway is impressive! With each consecutive pass my brain automatically makes a direct pathway! My verbal skills are finally, better than before, except when the human condition of nervousness crops up.

While I've been enhancing my brain, my ability to connect with people who are open and take responsibility for themselves, including their energy, continues to improve to deeper levels than before the TBI. Also, the visual image in my mind's eye of my journey to the lush green mountains has been fading.

In time, I will address the other areas in my brain that suffered brain damage. To be clear, I do not fix what is not broken, and I do not have delusional ideas of having a perfect memory or a super brain. This mind-set is foolish and is another reason why I will be very selective in whom I will teach.

Shortly after I completely healed my brain, I began approaching professionals and lay people (people with disconnections in their brain of all kinds, their families and friends, and the general public) to discuss and learn my method in person. But, no one is interested in learning or discussing my method or my new discoveries. Unfortunately, every person is locked in by *their* "No's and Never's," "Impossible's," negativity, and their focus on outside techniques. Rather than focus on what other people say and do. I choose to keep persevering, there have to be people in the world who want to learn my method, and or discuss my method. Hopefully in the future, people will be open.

It is summer 2000, and I take my time to fully enjoy all of my world-changing discoveries and accomplishments. I have a very strong gut sense that: exploring my brain from the inside, educating people from around the world, and working with professionals to research the brain and other ways to positively utilize my precise method will be a very wonderful lifelong journey.

34

THRIVING BETTER
THAN BEFORE

*Please note all of these jobs and activities are occurring during the same time frame.

While I am working full-time building log spiral stairs, I am also the Head Instructor teaching Kung Fu, a martial art, part time at the University of Colorado. I am responsible for seven to nine assistants and up to eighty-three students. I am also working on my own martial art training, and I am a positive asset to my friends, family, and community. On top of all that, I have a full social life, I love to hike, dance, travel, drive, read, cook, and of course, eat great food. I sleep between eight and nine hours a night and wake up refreshed. My life is extraordinarily rich and I treasure each and every moment!

First, I'll share how fate, in a round about way, planted the seed for my work of building log spiral stairs. A few years before I completely healed my brain, I was walking my dog Maja in an open field. Off in the distance was a shop that was building log stairs, railings, and more. I struck up a conversation with the two master craftsmen, who were really nice, and asked if I could look around. Happily, they said yes. I was in awe of the gorgeous stairs, the massive tools, and impressive woodworking shop. I was home; this was one of my dream jobs. At the time, I had no idea that, one day, my dream would come true.

The first day of building log stairs and more, I had to let go of my squared away, stick building, 2" x 4" world which I learned at North Bennett Street School in Boston and later honed in the working world. Each log stair I build is unique; nothing is square and nothing is perfectly round. The challenge of learning a whole new set of skills and language is invigorating. I am grateful that my learning curve is much faster because of my mind-set of *It's Easy* and of course, my precious inner awareness training. I am also fortunate to have an excellent teacher who is a master craftsman; he explains everything simply and clearly. I have a great deal of respect for my fellow craftsmen, my craft, and the humongous tools I use.

Building log spiral stairs from start to finish takes a tremendous amount of skill, and I love it! There are complex math problems that I solve, extensive organizational skills that I utilize to plan each one of a kind stair, and great physical strength needed to handle the XXXXL tools and logs wisely. I am constantly lifting between 20 lbs to over 100 lbs by myself. Since it's a very small shop, I am one of four people using timber carriers to lift and haul massive logs, and set up all kinds of stairs to be worked on.

There is also fine detail work in building log spiral stairs and straight run stairs. One of the tools I use is a log scriber. It takes a steady hand and a tremendous amount of hand-eye coordination to simultaneously focus on four points. The first two points are levels: one horizontal and one vertical. The third point follows the contour of the rough surface of the wood. The fourth point is the pencil that precisely marks the area to be cut out.

Another favorite task is making the flared root base for spiral stairs and posts. I thoroughly enjoy precisely marking and cutting a flat surface on the bottom of a log with its roots attached. I utilizing a multitude of equipment, here are a few. A transit helps to level the jigs that hold up the stair and posts. A laser light shows me the precise location of the bottom of the flared root base which I mark with a pencil. Next, I use a knife to cut into the wood which helps to avoid any splintering. Now, I am ready to use a chainsaw to cut the flared root base flat. To cut complex cuts – laps in post I use a massive 16" circular saw. This oversized saw is quite a change from the usual 7 ¼" used by carpenters.

My first attempt at making dovetails in the hand hewn balusters using a band saw is quite interesting to the say the least. Learning this task is like trying to shoot pool backwards, with a mirror, a warped cue, and a dangerous piece of equipment. Fortunately, making dovetails in the balusters quickly becomes second nature and it is a blast! This is a small sampling of what I do on a daily basis and the mammoth tools I work with.

While I am building each stair, I think of the people who will be using my stair. Kids will grow up playing on and around the log spiral stair, and people will have great conversations while looking at this absolutely stunning, practical piece of art. Many times, I want to pinch myself to see if I'm dreaming. I am getting paid to do what I love! I love working with wood, and even better, teaching Kung Fu at the university!

35

TEACHING
ONE OF MY LIFE'S
PASSIONS

In August 2002, I began teaching Kung Fu at the University of Colorado through the rec program. The first semester and a half, I am the Assistant Instructor. The next six years, I am the Head Instructor. I have come a long way from being told that "I could never, ever go to school" to teaching at a university! My life is off the charts awesome!

Intentionally, I have created a positive, healthy, encouraging class environment. We work hard, make great progress, and have a heck of a lot of fun. I have discovered that when people are having fun while working hard; they want to learn more and they are able to do so much more than they ever thought was possible.

Walking to my class at Carlson, the second oldest building at CU, I make sure my mind-set is squared away. My goal for each class is for it to be the best class ever, which elevates every class to a higher level. While setting up my class, I talk with my assistants and students as they come in and answer any questions. I am so very blessed to have phenomenal students and exceptional assistants, especially Paul "The Rock of Gibraltar" Smith and Robert Bowen. These two are my right hand assistants and trusted friends.

My class has people from around the country and around the world. I thoroughly enjoy meeting and getting to know people from different cultures and backgrounds; it makes my heart sing. What's interesting is in most martial art classes and schools there is usually a majority of male students. However, in my class there is more of a balance of male and female students, especially in the summer.

A few minutes before class begins, I gather my assistants. They are excellent martial artists and teachers who inspire me. Over time, we have built a very positive, healthy, strong connection. I share with them the things we will be working on which always includes having a great workout, making this the best class ever, and of course, having fun. *Experience has taught me that purposefully setting our mind-sets for the upcoming class raises our energy which is much more than physical. The powerful, uplifting energy invigorates us, flows through the class and students, and continues to thrive within many of us long after class ends. There are no words to explain this energy; it has to be personally experienced. It is especially important to purposefully make a decision and follow through with positive, healthy actions on days when I, or others, do not feel like training which is a natural part of working out. On these days, I consciously decide and enthusiastically tell my assistants that we are going to make this the best class ever, and again, we do!*

Class begins with a great warm up. While we are working out, I am aware of myself and how each student and assistant are doing with the conditioning and stretching, and as needed, I make adjustments.

I have transformed some of my brain healing techniques into teaching tools that are helpful to my students and assistants. Today, I am working with one of three white belt or beginner groups; there are ten people in each group. As I am teaching my white belt group, I am simultaneously making sure everything is going well with the seven other groups of students and assistants – from white belt through 1st Black. The total number of students for this class is eighty-three with seven assistants and my self. As I am teaching the techniques to the white belts, I am speaking the words for each movement out loud as if I am instructing a blind person or a person with disconnections in their brain. I am also making sure the students are following me correctly. I notice a few students giving me a weird look; I believe it's because I am speaking the movements out loud; regardless, I persevere.

After we have gone through the movements a few times, and I have answered all their questions, it's time for the students to give the movements a try on their own. They are doing pretty well; then, most of them get stuck, as usual, it is with those pesky transitional moves. Their frustration and confusion is clearly evident in their energy, body, and words. I have learned to wait for just the right moment, because if I explain my teaching tools too soon, students are not ready or motivated to put in the time and effort to get the results. When the students are ready, I share the story of speaking the movements out loud from my Simultaneous Brain Learning Method.

"In the beginning, no one believes speaking the movements loud enough to hear will work. Even I didn't believe it, until I tried it. Every person has sticking points in a form, and usually, it is with those pesky transitional moves. Now, not knowing what to do, whether in a martial art form or in life, has nothing to do with how smart you are or how much training you've had; it is a natural part of learning and life. It's what we do with these opportunities that make all the difference in the world.

Your brain is used to hearing your voice, tone, and choice of words, and it is definitely not used to my New England accent." The students smile. "I have discovered that speaking the movements loud enough to hear helps to get the movements, forms, and information deeper into the brain. I also know that it can be embarrassing to speak out loud, especially in front of a bunch of strangers. The first time, I used this technique I was embarrassed, and I was alone!" Everyone laughs.

"Even now, people will give me funny looks, and in the past, some people gave me a really hard time. But, I keep speaking the movements out loud because it works extraordinarily well. As for what words to say, that is a little bit of a challenge, in a good way. For now you can repeat my words, if you want. Later, you can change the words to whatever floats your boat.

Keep in mind, the only way you will really know that this technique or anything else works is by experiencing it for yourselves. If you are skeptical, remain skeptical. All I ask is that you be open, and as always, *give your absolute best effort with everything you do*. Any questions?" Everyone looks around, but no one speaks up.

"OK, we will go through these same movements a few more times while we are speaking the words for each movement out loud. Then, you will do the movements on your own. Alright, let's have some fun!"

While we are going through the form, I notice a little over half the students are speaking the words for the movements. When I finish teaching and answering questions, I calmly take a breath and in an instant deeply center myself and think, 'I *profoundly believe* that each student will own the movements they are working on!' I smile, look the students in the eye, and say with enthusiasm. "You are more than capable of doing all this and more! I have full confidence in you! You will own these movements by the end of class!" Each time, I profoundly believe in each student, then verbally express my sentiments that I absolutely know they will be successful; there is a positive shift in their energy and demeanor.

I watch the group perform the movements. The students who are speaking the movements out loud are improving at a much faster rate; it is a pure delight to watch the light bulbs go off. Some of them come up to me all excited, "I have improved more than I ever thought was possible! It really is much easier when

I speak the movements out loud while doing the moves!" "I am amazed how quickly I owned the movements!"

The students who were not saying the movements out loud observe for themselves the improvements in their fellow students. Many of them tentatively speak the movements out loud and their results are just as exceptional.

Before I teach the next set of moves, I compliment them on an excellent job. Many students who very much deserve the praise aren't able to accept my words. I explain. "Now, you do not know me. In time, you will figure out that I do not blow smoke / B.S., up anyone's pants, dress, shorts, gui, or anything else. When I give a compliment or tell you something works, I mean it."

A few minutes later, another assistant arrives from work, warms up, and asks how he can help. Since he is an excellent teacher, I have him work with the white belts; only the best people work with new students.

Now, I have eight assistants which provides me an opportunity to check in with all the other groups. While I am walking towards a more senior group of students, I see they are struggling to figure out the next move in a complex form, or more specifically, a section they were just taught. I bow to the assistant and patiently wait for the right moment. Without saying a word, I flick my right ear lobe and everybody smiles. They know that flicking the ear means; speak the movements loud enough to hear. Another way to get the point across is asking students while cupping my ear, "Have I gone deaf?" Being light hearted and having fun helps people to own whatever task their working on and sometimes it takes just a flick.

The students begin the section again while speaking the movements out loud, and easily flow past their sticking point, and finish the section. I give them a thumbs up and we smile. Before I move to the next group, I watch them give each other high fives and enthusiastically practice the section while speaking the words.

Students and assistants have integrated speaking the movements out loud and other techniques into their lives. Here is one story a student shared with me. "It was two o'clock in the morning, and I was studying for my biology test, my toughest class. I only had hours before the test, but no matter how hard I worked, I just kept struggling; the information was not getting into my brain. I was exhausted, discouraged, and all I wanted to do was sleep. Then, I heard your voice in my head. "Speak the words loud enough for you to hear!" I started saying the terms and definitions etc. out loud and everything began to make sense! I got so excited and even got my energy back! I wanted to let you know that I easily passed my biology test. Thank you for teaching me Kung Fu and for everything else!"

I firmly believe that people are more powerful and capable than they can imagine. The difficult and impossible becomes do-able by consistently making healthy decisions, relentlessly taking positive actions, and believing in oneself, another person, a horse, or a task, etc., and usually, the results far surpass what people could ever imagine.

On a regular basis, I relay to the class the success stories students and assistants have shared with me, whether in our Kung Fu class, their other classes, jobs, at home, and even in their businesses. Then, I remind them that although these techniques are great, they still have to go to class, study, do homework, etc. Everybody laughs.

The next story is how humor and being a little mischievous helps calm student's anxiety, especially white belts, before they test to their next belt level. I walk up to each white belt with a stern look on my face, and I have purposefully closed my body. They are shocked because usually I am smiling and have a great attitude. In a rigid tone and with my index finger following the beat of my words I say. "I am going to ask you the most important question I will ever ask." Each beginner student gets very nervous. I open my body and grin from ear to ear with this mischievous smile and cheerfully say, "What are you going to do to celebrate when you successfully pass your test?"

I love watching students smile and their entire being relax as they let out a huge sigh of relief. Some students ask how I know they are going to pass their test. My answer is simple. "I know you own your forms and you do them exceptionally well. But, there is much more to testing to your next belt level than owning forms. I have watched you from day one. You have had a great attitude, have consistently worked hard, and have unselfishly helped and encouraged others. It's a no-brainer; you will do well!"

What's interesting is after asking beginner students how they are going to celebrate, many times I have to wait for an answer because they are so taken aback by my question. I try to kick-start their thinking by asking if they are going to have a great meal, see a movie, or play video games. Sometimes, they still do not have an answer. I let them know that before they test, they will need to tell me how they are going to celebrate. Often, once students have had time to think about it, they enthusiastically say they are going to go for: an awesome hike, have a great dinner, hang out with friends and play video games, or go to a movie.

Quickly, it becomes a tradition for me to ask all students how they are going to celebrate successfully testing to their next belt level. To be clear, I only do the stern look thing for beginner students. The vast majority of mid-level and senior students see me walking up to them, and their smile gets bigger because they know what I am going to ask. I love that celebrating success has become a natural part of my class, and that people consciously choose to make each celebration more special. Sometimes I have not asked a student how they will celebrate successfully passing their test. The student seeks me out asking why I did not ask them the question. I apologize and ask. With glee they tell me this cool new way they are going to celebrate successfully passing their test.

The next story is about a student who decides to take a different direction. When I first started teaching at CU, I did not tell students about the TBI. However, after I became the Head Instructor, I shared that I completely healed my brain from a TBI and offered to teach everything I know about my method and the brain. As usual, I get the stunned looks and no-takers.

Considering my students know this information makes this next story a little bizarre, and in an unusual way, a high compliment.

Across the room I see Sally storming toward me. When she is a few feet away she loudly announces, "You have no idea how hard it is to remember these moves and these forms. I wish I had your memory." I look at her with compassion; this is not the first time a student has made this comment about my memory. However, memory is not this brilliant woman's problem. Sally expects to get the form the first time she sees it. My assistants and I have encouraged her to practice numerous times, but she will not put in the time and effort to practice during class or on her own. Instead of training, she watches other students do their forms.

I take a breath and ask Sally what form she is working on, and where are her sticking points. After she explains, we go through the section over and over again while I am speaking the movements out loud. I again ask her to speak the words, but she will not. As we are going through the section again, I stop just before one of her sticking points and ask, "What's the next move?" Sally is easily able to do the move, her sticking point, the next move, and the move after that.

We finish the section, and once again, I go over the techniques to improve memory: writing notes, visualization, speaking the movements out loud, along with other common sense techniques. I explain the upside and how easy and better it is to have a good work ethic which makes life and practicing forms so much easier and sweeter. I ask Sally if she understands and is willing to utilize these simple techniques. Without hesitating, she tells me that she understands, but she will not do the techniques. Her answer does not surprise me. I take a breath before responding.

"No one is able to master a form the first time they see it, and no one is able to be an expert if they do not put in the time and effort. You need to be willing to try and do *all* the work necessary to ingrain these movements in order to get *all* the results. The magic wand, plain and simple is – work. Having fun and a great attitude makes it so much sweeter and easier. Several times I have explained the different memory techniques and the reason to practice, but you will not use them and that is your choice.

As for me not knowing how hard it is to remember, you know I had a TBI. I have shared a few of the monumental stumbling blocks I faced and overcame. I did not wake up one morning and magically know how to completely heal my brain, how to own forms, and how to teach. I put in the time and effort to get all the results, and I had a blast doing it! So do not give me the line that I do not know how hard it is to remember.

Sally, it is easy to see that you are more than capable of physically doing the movements and mentally remembering them. But, you will not practice them and that is your prerogative. Success or failure rests squarely on your shoulders, not on anyone else's. When you are ready to put the time and effort in, I will be here. If you don't want to work with me, that's cool. You can work with one of my exceptional assistants."

Sally walks away and continues standing around watching other students train. Later, she comes up to me in a fury, repeating over and over again her negative mantra that I have no idea how hard it is to remember and she wishes she had my memory. Nothing I, or others, say can get through this woman's wall. Although Sally stops coming to class, my hope is one day she will stop being a "want to, want to," a person who wants the results, but will not do the work. In the future, when I am teaching my method, I will have 100% responsibility to choose my students, and I will be very wise in whom I select.

One of the things I love about my class is we are definitely not boring. We are always building upon what we have learned and changing what we are working on which greatly improves our growth. About a quarter of the way through this particular class, I ask the students to grab the thick shields and a partner. Grace, whom I would describe as petite, petite, asks Anne, a strong martial artist, who's about a foot taller, to hold the shield for her. Anne takes a sturdy stance and wraps the shield across her body. Each time Grace punches, she apologizes; even though, she is barely touching the shield.

Fast forward six months, and in this time we've probably done shield work five or six times. Grace is striking the shield and driving Anne back with ease, and Grace is not apologizing! Without saying a word, I motion to the other students and assistants to observe Grace. In awe, we watch this petite, petite woman easily uproot Anne! Step by step, Grace has experienced how to utilize her whole being and has far surpassed what she thought was possible.

People are more powerful when they focus their whole being. Once again, there are no limits or impossibilities, except in one's mind, which brings up my next point. In my class and in my life, the word *can't* is not allowed. I ask students to change their words to *I am not able to yet, I am working towards owning this section or form. Or other words that work for them.* In addition, no one is allowed to put down or make fun of anyone or anything, including themselves.

As often as I can, I tell my assistants and students how much I appreciate them. At the end of each class, I walk to the door and shake the hand of each student and assistant and thank them for: attending class, congratulate them on specific improvements that they have made during class, and / or for successfully testing. I also offer words of encouragement. My students and assistants inspire me as they continue to improve, grow, and change in and out of class.

For years, my class has grown by leaps and bounds. I believe our extraordinary success is a result of the positive way we teach, the conscious, healthy atmosphere we create, and how we conduct ourselves – more than the martial art we teach. On a regular basis, more people ask to attend my class, and students ask for more time to train because they are having so much fun learning and working out. What a wonderful blessing! Thankfully, semester after semester, my boss has increased the class size, from fifty three students to its current *eighty-three students.* To put this into perspective an average class size in this genre is between *thirteen and eighteen students.*

After a few years, my boss agrees to extend the class time from

1 ½ hours to 2 hours. Even with the extra half hour, students continue to enthusiastically ask for more time. Instead of asking for more time from my boss, which I know is not going to happen. We do what we have done for years. After class, we move our training upstairs in the hallway and practice until hunger pangs, or other pressing activities beckon us to stop teaching.

What is really interesting is after class, a few of my assistants and I will either do our own martial art training or we will hang out with other martial artists who are training. Something really, really strange happens; actually, it's been happening since I became the Head Instructor. The other martial artists are always in super, super slow motion: physically and verbally. My assistants and I try to explain what is occurring to the other martial artists, but they do not understand. What is interesting is that when my assistants and I are not coming from teaching at CU, our martial art friend's speech and actions are at their normal speed. Instead of continuing to explain what is happening, my assistants and I decide to simply enjoy this magnificent palpable energy. I believe our experience is, again, a result of purposefully having a positive mind-set and elevating ourselves and our energy before each class, which again is much more than physical. To truly understand this phenomenon, a person needs to experience it for them self.

I am very blessed and honored to be a part of our class. This very special time and place has been given to us to enjoy, grow, and thrive as martial artists, and more importantly, as human beings. My students and assistants have taught me so much, and for that, I am extraordinarily thankful. My hope is to always have a student mind-set, to strive for excellence – not perfection, and to enjoy each moment. I believe that what I have learned from teaching Kung Fu at the university, and all my other experiences in life has prepared me to teach my Brain Phoenix ™ method.

36

IT'S GOOD TO
HAVE
PERSPECTIVE

The vast majority of people who knew me while I had a TBI, and now that I have completely healed and enhanced my brain are ecstatic and are very proud of all my accomplishments and success. Though, there are a few people who try to use the former TBI to their advantage. These two stories reveal how other people think and feel about themselves.

When my job changed from the Assistant Instructor to the Head Instructor of Kung Fu at the university, I became a target of a small group of martial artists who have a penchant for trying to discredit and bully people, and intentionally cause all kinds of strife. The more successful I am, especially with my class, the more determined they are to put me down as a martial artist, instructor, and human being. Though sometimes it gets to me, the one thing I can control is my reaction. I consciously choose not to focus on what they say and do. Again, their words and actions are announcing to the world how they think and feel about themselves, not anyone else. Years pass, and despite all their attempts to cause trouble, or as I like to say, their negative energy gunk, my class continues to prosper. Then, they decide to go after the one thing they think will break me.

Robert Bowen, one of my trusted assistants pulls me aside. I can tell he wants to talk, but he is nervous. Finally he says, "Cathy, you know (he names the martial artists in the bullying group) how they are always spreading nasty rumors and purposefully doing everything they can to put you and other people down and causing all kinds of discord?" He hesitates. "Well, they are saying that you never had a TBI, that you do not have any signs of brain damage, and that you are just looking for sympathy. They are telling people not to believe you when you say you had a TBI."

Robert thinks I am going to be really upset. He is shocked when I let out a huge belly laugh! I am laughing so hard, I am doubled over grabbing my knees, and having a hard time catching my breath. Tears of laughter are flowing down my face. (In fact, I am laughing as I write this.) After a few minutes, I catch my breath and say. "They have no idea what a massive compliment they gave me! This is their pinnacle of put downs! That's not a put down, that's a phenomenal off the charts compliment!"

I have discovered that people are more afraid of being successful than they are of failure. The more negative – fearful a person is, the more likely they will disparage themselves, others, and organizations, etc. whether it is through snide remarks, gossip, or outright destructive acts.

What is interesting is that other people who know about the bullying situation tell me to just shrug it off. But, when those same bullies go after them, they do not understand. I share with them that I can empathize. But, they get pissed off and indignantly say, "Yea, but that's happening to you. You do not understand this is happening to me!" I quickly reply, "It's okay that the bullies were and are going after me, but now that it is happening to you, it's not okay?" He stumbles in his response,

"Yes! Well, well, no. But, but, but you know what I mean." I inhale and say, "Not cool dude. Not cool."

The next story, I call a *label of convenience.* I am having a blast practicing a whole bunch of upper Black Belt forms on my own, and I am enjoying an excellent workout. In the middle of a form, I notice two fellow Black Belts, Angelina and Tad, a wife and husband, intensely watching me. They were great supporters when I had the TBI. Since I have completely healed and enhanced my brain, Angelina continues to treat me extremely well, as she does everyone else. Tad, on the other hand, has had a rather difficult time making the transition.

I finish a form, and I am about to start another form when Tad says, "We've been real busy with work and that's why we haven't been around." I smile and say, "It's good to see you both." Tad asks, "The last form you did was that Tiger / Crane?" My smile widens, "Yes, Tiger / Crane is so much fun! I love the dynamic power, rooting, and flow of the tiger, and the graceful, lightning fast, pinpoint strikes of the crane!" Tad hesitantly says, "Well ahh, we're getting ready to test, and we need to get the Tiger / Crane form down. Would you help us get the Tiger / Crane form?" "Sure, let's go"

While going through the Tiger / Crane form, I am speaking the words for each movement out loud and spending extra time on those pesky transitional moves. What is shocking is that Tad is interacting with me as an equal. However, once he owns the form, his entire demeanor changes. Within his thank you is an attempt to put me into the prison of less than. "Well, thanks for all your help. Your head must be hurting and you must be tired. You should rest. We know you have a difficult time remembering things."

I look him square in the eye. I have just finished reviewing an advanced Black Belt form. I was absolutely thorough in my teaching, my memory was impeccable, and I explained the movements and transitional moves exceptionally well. I also treated them with respect and as an equal. I become aware that my back is rearing up. Fortunately, I prayed beforehand and compassion washes over me. I take a deep breath, smile, and say. "My head is fine since I have completely healed my brain. In fact, I have so much energy that I am going to do a whole bunch of advanced black belt forms. Do you want to join me?" I smile. I am okay that a little bit of smart-ass came out while speaking. Tad answers, "Oh no, we have to be going. You know, we are really busy."

Negative people are trying to nurture their hungry souls with the very thing that is starving them – their own fear. They are choosing to be enmeshed in their fear, plummeting backwards, and believing that if they put others and even themselves down, they will become powerful and feel better about themselves and their lives. But, their negativity always boomerangs and rips deeper into their embattled souls. When people try to confine, define, or control others or a situation, they are afraid – fear is their driving force. Once again, their negative, fear-filled words, actions, and energy are announcing to the world how they think and feel about themselves, not anyone or anything else.

Every human being wants and needs to be loved, accepted, and respected. The negative, fear-filled people are looking for relief on the outside, when the solution always begins inside – their thinking. Every person is an expert at persevering, and each moment, we make a decision to persevere forwards; flowing with the stream of life, or persevere – move backwards; flowing against life. There is only one thing we human beings can truly control or direct – our thinking. Some people say that it is too hard to change their thinking and life. My experience, and I have had a lot of it, is that it is easier and a heck of a lot less work to persevere forwards and to have a positive attitude by consistently making healthy decisions, taking positive actions, being responsible for oneself, and repeating.

37

THE ONLY PLACE IMPOSSIBLE RESIDES IS IN THE MIND, BUT NOT IN MINE

Soon after I completely healed my brain, I began another journey offering to discuss and teach my precise method – in time I will call it Brain Phoenix ™, to doctors, scientists, researchers, and lay people (people with intact brains, people with disconnections in their brain of all kinds [brain problems], their families and friends, and the general public). I share how the method I developed completely healed my brain from a TBI, some of my accomplishments, and my goal of teaching my method and everything I know about the brain to people throughout the world. It is paramount for students to be studied and tested before, during, and after they have completed my method. My primary focus is to teach people to become instructors. After students have completed the whole process; then, received their teaching degree, my hope is they will go back to their state or nation, and using the same high standards, will teach others how to completely heal and enhance the brain. One of my motivations for teaching is that I do not want others to suffer as I did, disconnected and imprisoned in the brain. It's time to turn hopelessness into hope.

To my surprise, there are **three distinct reactions**, and over time, it becomes even more informative. Although I am **simultaneously** approaching professionals and lay people – to make it clearer, I will summarize the reactions into three separate groups – (1) professionals, (2) people with disconnections in their brain, and (3) their families and friends and the general public.

(1) Professionals. I introduce myself to each professional explaining that I had a TBI and have developed a precise method that completely healed my brain. I share a little bit about my method, some of my accomplishments, and my goals. Silence. For ten to fifteen seconds every professional is stunned. After gathering their composure, each professional gently escorts me out their office without saying a word, and the door slams in my face. Some people have thrown me out mid-sentence. Through the door, I thank each professional for their time. My mind-set is every person and organization that says no, means I am one step closer to people saying yes. After many, many negative experiences, I catch myself muttering as I walk away from the door of another professional, "You snooze, you lose." Though it temporarily takes some of the sting away, it is an immature, negative attitude. I need to transform my mind-set.

This calling has chosen me and it is bigger than me. What other people think, say, and do is none of my business. I will keep persevering and succeed in my endeavor to teach my method to people throughout the world. Next, I ask friends and mentors for suggestions on how to improve my approach with the professionals. They put my naiveté and the professionals' reactions into perspective. Here is one which pretty much sums up all of their suggestions. "Cathy, we know you are an honest person, but those professionals do not know you. When you say you have developed a precise method that completely healed your brain to a neurologist, neuro-psychologist, neuro-scientist, etc., it's like telling an oncologist that a juice drink will cure cancer. Yes, they could have been professional, but they weren't. Cathy, move on. You have to keep trying; so many people need your help."

There is an additional, noteworthy comment made by friends and mentors who have a master's degree and higher. They suggest when I speak and write about my approach and interactions with professionals and their organizations to downplay what happened, because in the future I will be teaching them, and they will be working for and with me.

I reflect on the changes I want to make in my approach with professionals, and I also take into account my friends' suggestions. I make three decisions. First, I will adjust my approach with professionals by ending my summary that I was the one who had a TBI. Second, after each conversation I will contemplate what happened and make changes to my approach, if appropriate. Third, from this point forward, when I discuss, teach, or speak about my method, I will only name the professionals, their organizations, and the lay people who were respectful.

(2) People with disconnections in their brain. While I am approaching professionals, I am **simultaneously** reaching out to people with disconnections in their brain. Their reactions are completely different than the professionals. Each person listens intently as I describe my previous brain damage, deficits, the years at rehab, and trying to make my brain smart by going to college. Next, I talk about my method, a few of my accomplishments, and desire to teach my method. **I am flabbergasted – Each person who has enough verbal wherewithal keeps asking, "How do you know about the prison in *my* brain."**

Again, I share that I was able to touch the prison wall in my brain and pound on it with all my might with my fists and forearms, but I did not have the power to break through. The world I lived in my entire life had become a foreign outside world. Inside my brain, I experienced a depth of utter loneliness and agony unlike anything I'd ever known. There was also a sense of peace inside my brain, but it was insignificant compared to the loneliness and agony. There are no words to describe the profound sense of losing connection with everyone and everything, including my own body. The farther away a body part was from the prison in my brain, the more disconnected it was. My brain did not know where my feet were, even though I could see them. Everything outside the thick, blurry glass prison, including my own body, was a foreign outside world. Before the TBI, I had great hand, eye, and body coordination; afterwards, I was beyond awkward. Initially, I did not understand why the people in the foreign outside world could not see me in my brain and break me out. I did not know why I was locked in my brain and why it was so difficult to get information into and out of the thick, blurry glass wall. I finally accepted that other people and anything outside of me did not have the power and the tools to liberate me. *While I am speaking, each person's face and eyes light up, and their heads are nodding up and down. Next, I once again share about my precise method, accomplishments, and goal of teaching my method. In mid-sentence each person dramatically stops me, leans way in with their arms and hands reaching as if to grab me. The people with the verbal wherewithal ask over and over again. "How do you know? How do you know about the thick, blurry, glass prison in **my brain**? How do you know?"*

*At first, I am taken aback. No one has spoken to them about being imprisoned in their brain. Then, I realize that it was only after I liberated myself that I was able to talk about my past experience of the thick, blurry glass prison. I change my approach in how I explain the TBI, the prison wall that was in my brain, and my method. Impulsively, they tell me, in no uncertain terms, that they understand my method and what I did, but they really do not care about that. All they want to know is, "How do you know about the prison in **my brain**?" Again, I* *change my approach, but they continue asking over and over. "How do you know about the prison in **my brain?**"*

*Every explanation and offer to teach my method is dismissed. But, they continue asking, "How do you know about the prison in **my** brain?" I take a breath. This is not about disconnections in the brain; it's about closed minds. Exasperated, and right on cue, they tell me they have already accepted that there is no hope of recovery for them. All the doctors and therapists have pounded that into them. My heart aches as, one by one, people say, over and over again. "I will never, ever be healed, so what's the use in trying." It is disheartening listening to all their "Can'ts," "No's and Never's," "Impossibles," and plethora of excuses. Nothing I say can get through their closed mind-sets. Compassion wells within me. They have made their decision and have accepted their permanent internment; even though, I know there is a solution to completely liberate themselves from the prison in their brain.*

I believe the agony of being imprisoned in the brain does not even come close to consciously choosing to be utterly hopeless. I am grateful that I did not accept the TBI, other's "impossible's" "no's and never's," and negativity. I take a breath and thank each person for their time. I need to find people with open minds, who want to be free, who trust my method will work for them, and who are committed to do *all* the work to get *all* the results.

(3) Families and friends of people with disconnections in their brains and the general public. While I am reaching out to professionals and people with disconnections in their brain, I am **simultaneously** approaching family members and friends of people with disconnections in their brain, and the general public. I give my quick summary of my brain healing journey, the precise method I developed that completely healed my brain, a few of my accomplishments, and desire to teach my method. Silence. For ten to fifteen seconds people are stunned. They lean in, search deep into my eyes, and stare at my face. After they gather their composure, most of them say. "Cathy, if you had not told me, I would have never known you had a TBI. There are no signs of brain damage on your face, in your eyes, or on your body, and your speech is eloquent. Are you a doctor or a scientist?"

"No." "Well, you need to write a book about your life and your extraordinary method. You will help so many people, and I will be the first one to buy your book! Of course, you are going to need an M. D. and or a celebrity's name on the cover to promote you and your book."

I smile and gently say, "Writing a book is the last thing I want to do. My goal is to teach my method and everything I have discovered in the brain to as many people throughout the world. I am a very private person; I do not want notoriety. I would rather be digging ditches in the rocky soil of New England, in the middle of winter, during a Nor'easter, than write a book about myself." *What I do not say is that if I wrote a book, it would have to be thousands and thousands of pages long to explain everything I did to completely heal and enhance my brain, but that would still be incomplete because my method needs to be taught in person.*

I continue, "As for needing a doctor to legitimize my method that does not make sense." I reiterate, "I have not been able to get professionals or anyone else to discuss or learn my method. My method is not about me or anyone else; my method is about helping others."

Over and over again, people say that I need to keep reaching out to others and that what I have done is a miracle. I explain that it was not a miracle; I absolutely needed to discover a way to liberate myself in order to be reconnected. People change directions; instead of talking about my method or taking me up on my offer to learn my method; they, once again, try to convince me of the necessity of a person who carries weight to get my message across. Again, I explain the challenges of getting people to listen and discuss my method, never mind taking me up on the offer to learn it. I steer the conversation back to my method, but they change the subject and talk about anything else. I do not understand why people will not take advantage of this phenomenal opportunity to discuss the brain, my precise method, and or learn my method.

What is fascinating and frustrating is that the vast majority of people's energy, body language, and words match up – they believe what I am saying and they want me to succeed. But, they also have this conflicting energy like they do not know they can talk about the brain or how to talk about the brain. I get the sense that they think it is sacrilege to talk about the brain. The more I talk about the brain and my method, the taller and thicker they build their walls; it's like their putting up two huge hands to stop. I decide to keep my comments about the brain to a bare minimum, but even that seems to be too much for everyone; including professionals. It is beyond frustrating not having anyone to talk with about my method and all my phenomenal discoveries.

People continue talking about everything else except my method. Instead of going down that road, I make the best out of each opportunity. I ask if they know of any professionals or lay people who would be interested in learning and discussing my method, and if they have any other suggestions. There is a sense of discouragement in their energy, being, and voices, almost always they say no; the people they know will not listen. I thank them for their time. I reach out to the few people that have been suggested; unfortunately, it is more closed minds. Wow, I thought reaching out and teaching my method would be a breeze; it may be more challenging.

(1) Next, I try a new approach with *other* professionals. Now, I am speaking even faster than my rapid pace of New Englandese, because I do not know how long before a door might slam in my face. Usually after thirty seconds to one minute, I am almost always asked, "Are you a doctor or a scientist?" When I answer no, it's obvious my status had been downgraded, and my time has been greatly reduced. Confidently I continue; then, conclude by saying that I was the one who had a TBI, and I developed my precise method that completely healed my brain.

Every professional is stunned and absolutely silent for ten to fifteen seconds. They lean in, peer deep into my eyes and face; it's like their minds are in hyper drive. They gather their composure, sit straight up, and most of them indignantly say that I am not a doctor or a scientist so how could I know what I was talking about. They conclude that it is impossible to heal the brain. I politely thank each professional; then, take time to reflect on each experience. They were respectful and dealt with me as an equal while I was articulating my method, up until I said I was not a doctor or a scientist. After disclosing that I was the one who had the TBI, they dropped me from second class to fourth class. Unfortunately, these experiences remind me of an incident that occurred shortly before I completely healed my brain.

Prior to breaking through the thick, blurry glass wall, I knew it was only a matter of time and effort before I completely healed my brain. Since I am not a scientist, I believed professionals needed to verify my progress and test my method in order for the process to be duplicated. However, the window to study and test me was closing very quickly. I called my neurologist, but he had retired. Although I was very hesitant to make an appointment with the new doctor, the drive to help other people liberate themselves pushed any uncertainty aside.

The appointment with the new neurologist was going very well. He listened, asked pertinent questions, and I answered his questions correctly. I continued to be very cautious to speak about my goal of completely healing and enhancing my brain better than before, my precise method so far, and all the progress I had made. Nevertheless, I needed to step up – other people's freedom depended on it. "I am developing a method to completely heal my brain and I am making phenomenal progress. I believe I need help to test and document my." In mid-sentence he interrupted me and exploded into a complete rage. He said that it was impossible to heal the brain and pointed out that without a medical degree I knew nothing. His fury continued to build. Pure contempt exuded from his being. His body language was rigid, and the expressions on his face were shock and disdain. I pleaded with him to test and document my progress and method so others could be helped. He bolted from his chair, leaned against the counter a few feet away, crossed his arms and legs, and yelled even louder; then, he laughed at me. Nothing I said could persuade him. He continued to loudly belittle and laugh at me as I rose from the chair, crossed the threshold, closed the door behind me, and walked down the hallway. I was crushed. His utter disrespect and unprofessional conduct astounded me.

In time, my friends and mentors helped me to look at this experience in a different light. "This was the first time you had met him. He did not know that you are a person of integrity who has been working really hard for a long time. He also did not know all the progress you made because he did not give you the opportunity. Yes, he could have listened, and yes, he should have been professional, but that is not what happened. *He is responsible for his words and actions.* Keep moving forward Cathy, so many people need your help."

Reflecting on this past experience and my recent attempts to talk with professionals helps me to put everything into perspective. I did not let that doctor stop me, and I will not let anyone stop me. I need to keep persevering; people's freedom is on the line. However, from this point forward, I will not tell professionals about the TBI whom I approach about my method.

I continue reaching out to professionals and lay people, but **no one wants to discuss or learn my method**. Again, people talk about everything else except my method. Once more, exuding from their bodies when I talk about the brain and my method is this conflicting energy like they do not know they can talk about the brain or how to talk about the brain. I share with my friends and mentors about the recent experiences and ask for suggestions. Unfortunately, I have already tried what they have proposed without any success. They ask if I am ready to contact N.E.R.H. (New England Rehabilitation Hospital) I tell them no; the possibility of being rejected by the people who were so wonderful to me, especially Dr. Peterson, would be too much to bear.

When I become the head instructor of Kung Fu at C.U., I switch my approach with professionals, and everything changes. Now, I introduce myself as a martial art instructor, I have developed a method and have taught a woman with a TBI how to completely heal her brain. All of what I say is true. I taught myself and I developed my method. Next, I give a quick explanation of my method, and the need to teach, study, test, and research people. Each professional listens intently; their energy and bodies are open, and when I finish speaking they too are stunned. The usual ten to fifteen seconds passes. Then, in a respectful manner, they ask if I am a doctor or a scientist. To my surprise and delight, when I answer no, they continue to communicate with me as a fellow professional. Again, I talk about my desire to teach people, to study, and test my method. Their energy completely changes. Their dejected responses are very informative. "I do not have the power to make decisions. You need to talk with my boss or his boss."

I am shocked! I always thought neurologists, neuroscientist, neuro-psychologists, physiatrists, other doctors, therapists, etc. are people with power. Even within medicine and science, there is a hierarchy of power. My heart goes out to these professionals. They work diligently and really want to help their patients, but their hands are tied. Although I do not understand why they will not talk about the brain, my discoveries and method, I accept their decision. I profoundly express my appreciation for their attentiveness and professionalism. Next, I talk with or attempt to talk with their bosses, but once again, all the pathways are dead-ends. I ask myself, 'Who has the power? I need to find the people with power.'

(2 and 3) My approach also changes when I meet lay people. Instead of immediately talking about me and my method, I take the time to get to know people, especially what makes their heart sing. I have consciously chosen for them to get to know me – as the person I am now – without labels. I do not tell people right away that I had a TBI because it would be really awkward, like TBI is a natural part of a conversation. If they ask what I do and if it's appropriate, I give a quick summary of my experience, my method, some of my accomplishments, and desire to teach and research. The response of families and friends, and the general public is pretty much the same; no one wants to learn or talk about my method. However, there are rare occasions when a

family member asks how much it will cost to learn my method. I tell them I have not gotten that far because no one has stepped up, but we can talk about it. Rather than discuss how much it will cost, they completely change the subject. Also, a few people have asked if my method will work for everyone. My answer is simple; no. Students need to believe they will be completely healed and they must be able to complete my whole method – do *all* the work, to get *all* the results. Students need to be enthusiastic about learning my whole method and helping others. (Shortly, I will clearly state the requirements for students, staff, and organizations.) As usual, instead of discussing my method etc., people change the subject.

Another response from some family members is they continue asking me to talk with their loved ones with disconnections in their brain; even though, I have already tried, and they have declined to discuss and learn my method. My powerful past has taught me that it is futile to keep approaching the same people and try to break through their closed mind-sets. Trying to shove something down a person's throat is a good way to get them throwing up on your shoes, meaning: get resentful, mouthy, and balk. *It's their job to open their minds, not mine.*

In addition, when it comes to the brain, some people need to complicate things. In my experience, while in the process of developing my method it was imperative to keep things simple. I needed to get down to the bare basics of what worked, what didn't work, and why. Of the utmost importance was to always delve deeper into my precious inner awareness training. If I had complicated things, there is no doubt I would still be imprisoned in my brain. The outside intellectual information of making neural connections, being shown the plastic brain model with the removable lobes, and where the damage occurred in my brain was only helpful **after I discovered a way to enter my brain.**

I am at the point that closed minds and rejections from professionals and lay people do not bother me. I decide to contact Dr. Peterson and the wonderful people at N.E.R.H. (New England Rehabilitation Hospital) Hopefully, they will choose to discuss and / or learn my method. I am told Dr. Peterson has retired, and she and her husband have gone to Africa to help people. As for other doctors and therapists at rehab who helped me, I am not given the opportunity to approach them. Though I am surprised, and a bit disappointed, I do not kick my butt; that would be a total waste of time and effort. I accept that at this time it was not meant to be, and I will continue to try to find Dr. Peterson and others.

(While writing this book I am given Dr. Peterson's email address. By email I thanked her for how well she treated me, and for being an exceptional doctor and human being. I wrote that I had developed a, step by step, method that completely healed my brain. I also shared some of my accomplishments and included photos. I expressed a great willingness to explain my method in detail via the internet, in person, or whatever was convenient for her. We emailed back and forth several times over the course of many months. My offer has not been accepted – yet. In the future, I look forward to Dr. Peterson and the other exceptional team members *meeting me with an intact brain*. I want to thank them in person, and explain my method that completely healed an enhanced my brain better than before the TBI.)

(1 and 3) I continue reaching out to other professionals, family members and friends of people with disconnections in their brain, and the general public, though the experiences are the same. Again, the vast majority of people are intrigued, but they are conflicted about talking about the brain and my method.

(2) On the other hand, the reactions of people with disconnections in their brain are very informative. Here are more experiences. While briefly explaining my previous brain damage, deficits, rehab, school, and my method, people listen intently. Though there have been a few who become totally enraged – fearful when I say the word *meditation*. Their energy closes, their faces scrunch up, and their arms and legs cross as they angrily say. "Meditation is a new age or religious thing. If I have to meditate, I will not do your method."

Gently, I explain, "The way I utilized meditation had nothing to do with new age or religion. Meditation is focused thinking. If you have ever worried about a problem or a situation – you have meditated. If you have focused on a task, a word, or a phrase, then you can meditate. If you have been aware of your breath or heartbeat, you have meditated. Meditation improves focus and energy which is a really good thing.

Some other benefits of meditation are increasing oxygen levels, relieving stress, and centering one-self. What's great is that once you own the basic principles of meditation, it's rather easy and simple to do basic meditation, and you can practice wherever and whenever you want. I meditated with a TBI and if I can meditate, anyone can. If you're skeptical about meditation, I encourage you to remain skeptical, and be open." Unfortunately, many people are so ticked off that they abruptly walk away.

The next story is about a person with a TBI who is in the process of getting on Social Security Disability Insurance (S.S.D.I.). He explains that he cannot do my method because if he gets better, he will not get on S.S.D.I., and he does not know how to pay for the bare necessities of rent, food, and medical insurance. What he says is true, if he gets even a little better he might not qualify for S.S.D.I. Other people on S.S.D.I. have expressed the same sentiment; a person does not have to be completely healed to lose their benefits. I explain that I too was afraid of losing my benefits while I was developing my method. However, I kept persevering because I had to liberate myself in order to be reconnected. Unfortunately, people continue focusing on *their* "Impossible's," "No's and Never's," and their long list of excuses and negativity.

Hopefully in the future, people will open their minds, and they will not lose their benefits while going through the process of completely healing and enhancing their brains. Solutions need to be in place so people can focus on healing, rather than be stressed over finances and insurance. But, **freedom isn't free.** *Although I do not have any answers to this issue, my focus must be on teaching and continuing my brain research and other research.*

There's another response I hear over and over again from

people with disconnections in their brain. They need *relief* and they are seeking it in all sorts of ways. Here are some of the things people have done and are doing. Vitamins, yoga, hiking, biking, reading, listening to music, playing an instrument, trying to write songs, juice drinks, eating different foods, and even boxing. I ask each person, "Have you received the relief you are looking for?" They sigh and share, "I get some relief, but it is never enough. Do you know of a brain supplement, food, or a quick brain healing technique that will help me?" While others say, "All I want is a magic pill or wand to fix me." When a person wants a quick brain healing technique or magic wand etc. this is a huge red flag.

I share about eating and sleeping well, working out regularly, and equally important, being aware of one's thinking. A much easier and more enjoyable way of living is to flow with life by being positive and persevering forwards. Next, I reiterate that no one and nothing from the foreign outside world could break through the thick, blurry glass prison that was in my brain. There wasn't a magic pill or wand. The relief and freedom I was seeking had to come from inside me, which it did. Again, I try to explain that I teach a precise three phase, step by step, method that completely healed my brain. Once again, they say they totally understand what I did; even though, they have not let me fully explain my method. Their energy and voices changes to dejection; in barely a whisper they say a very familiar phrase, "I can't be free. It's impossible, so why try."

Some people try to brush me off by saying that I don't know how hard they have it. I share a few of the challenges I have faced, overcome, and that I'm thriving. Their eyes open wide, and they change their pissing contest mentality. "You're a strong, courageous person, and I'm not. I couldn't do what you've done." Quickly I respond, "Courage is not being free of fear. Courage is stepping up despite what other people think, say, and do. Courage is saying frig the fear and doing what needs to be done. Every person is courageous inside, and it's a conscious choice to tap into this power or not. I walked through the fear because I got so damn tired of people trying to beat me down with *their* negativity, "impossible's," and "no's and never's." I needed to be free, and I did whatever it took to liberate and reconnect myself." Next, they tell me that they don't have time to do my method. I ask, "What do you do?" Their answer does not surprise me. "Not much." Again, they focus on all the things they can't do and won't ever be able to do. I thank each person for their time and keep moving forward.

The years pass and I have approached thousands and thousands of people, but every path is a dead-end. People's mind-set reminds me of the belief that the world is flat, always has been flat, and will always be flat. I want to clap my hands and yell, Wake up! But I don't because that would be a waste of time and effort. This part of my journey, approaching professionals and lay people, is light years more challenging than it was to discover, develop, and successfully implement my method – Brain Phoenix ™.

If a person had talked with me, or I had heard about a method that completely healed the brain while I had the TBI, I would have wanted to know everything there is about the brain and their method. I would have asked pertinent questions, and listened as intently as I could in order to make an informed decision. I would have brought along wise professionals and lay people with intact brains, and asked them to ask insightful questions and to discuss this method at length.

My family, friends, and lay people bluntly tell me. "Just give up. If people want to stay imprisoned in their brains, and or have closed minds, so be it. You have gone above and beyond what anyone would expect you to do."

Should I give up and say the heck with peoples: negativity, "No's and Never's," "Impossible's," and excuses? I remind myself that *the biggest obstacle a person will ever face is their own thinking, and the easiest thing to change is one's thinking. It begins by making one healthy decision, taking positive actions, and repeating.*

An interesting thing happens every time I think about ending my journey to teach and discuss my method. I see a person who has disconnections in their brain, and most of the time they are with their family and friends. Emanating from them is a sense of long term despair, mixed with positive and negative energy and emotions. The first few times this happened I was surprised, though each time it helps me to pause and reflect.

Every time I have thought about giving up, my thinking was ruled by frustration and doubt – fear; a clear indication that I had gotten off my path. To get back on track, I decide to focus on and feed my passions for this journey. Here are a few. I do not want others suffering as I did, disconnected and imprisoned in the brain. This calling is bigger than I, and bigger than anyone and anything else. This is *all* about my method – Brain Phoenix ™; it is not about me, an individual, a group, or an organization, or anything else. I believe there are people in the world who want to be free and reconnected. I remind myself that the only place impossible resides is in the mind, but not in mine, and hopefully not in others. I decide to continue approaching professionals and lay people and offering to teach and discuss my method.

38

LOVE AND
SUPPORT
2005

For years, I have had a dream and have been making plans to open two schools. My main focus is my Brain Phoenix ™ school, teaching my method to people from around the world, and also a Kung Fu School in Hawaii. It is spring, and although things are blossoming; it also feels like everything is coming to a close in Colorado. I start thinking about making a huge leap of faith; selling my home and putting my plans into action.

In an instant, our lives can turn upside down, and there is nothing we can do to prevent these tough times. People think it will not happen to them, but it happens to everyone: loss of job, relationship, friends, accident, illness, medical tests (waiting for and hearing the results), and of course, death. These are a few things people will experience personally or with a loved one. It's not *if* these things will happen; it's *when*.

In June 2005, out of nowhere the cancer returns and this time it is aggressive. Dr. Kearsey, an oncologist, tells me the treatments are going to be hard. I'm in professional athlete shape. I know what hard is; I can handle it. I put everything on hold, and immediately begin chemo. Rather quickly, I lose all my muscle mass and vitality. Simply lifting my arm feels like I'm trying to drag it through thick, wet, cold concrete. Hard, I thought I knew what physically hard was; I did not have a clue.

The mind games one plays after getting diagnosed with cancer or other massive life altering challenges are rather interesting. One question that is dominating my thinking is; What could I have done to prevent the cancer? Although science does not have a definitive answer, I decide to examine where I was at mentally, emotionally, physically etc. right before the cancer began.

I ask Dr. Kearsey when did the cancer return; taking into account the cat scans and other tests? She contemplates the question and says about six months ago. I go into reflection mode. During that time, I was very afraid of losing my job. The next thought slowly drifts in. It was the dead of winter, and I thought it would be difficult to find a carpentry or woodworking job. How would I pay my mortgage and bills? I shake my head and start kicking my butt for being so foolish. Consciously, I chose to travel backwards and had knowingly fed the fear. Seconds later, I stop mentally kicking my butt. I know full well this negative path is a colossal waste of time and effort. I refuse to go backwards and flow against life – that is nuts.

I make a decision that turns my thinking around. I refuse to allow fear to rule my thinking and life. From this point forward, I will not feed the fear of losing jobs, money, or other B.S. I will not crash and burn about money. Being human, I know fear will crop up, and it will come in all sorts of shapes and sizes – negative thinking gunk. Instead, I will consciously feed and trust my faith, and I will follow my gut – *no matter what.*

Next, my focus shifts to the fact that I was in phenomenal shape before the diagnosis. Though, the past year plus, I let my internal training; meditation, chi kung postures, Tai Chi, Pa Kua, Hsing I, etc. slack big time. I dig a little deeper and look at my mind-set. With **all** the internal work I had done and **all** the progress I had made, I thought I was set for life. Look at how far I have come; I do not have to practice on a regular basis. After all, I know how to completely heal and enhance the brain. I laugh at my immature, arrogant attitude. **Well, La Ti Friggin Da!** My negative, unhealthy thinking is similar to the belief that working out once or eating one meal should last a lifetime. Although I said my health was important, my actions spoke louder than my words. Though I was in phenomenal shape before the cancer, I could have done a lot better, from the inside out.

My mind totally shifts gears. In spring 2001, I had had an accident; my small truck (not the big ole ass truck) was totaled by a reckless driver. *I hit my head and something familiar happened. Over the next few days, I had this intense need to sleep and was powerfully drawn to go toward the same wonderful, peaceful, warm water and beach that I experienced right after the TBI. Again, I was at a crossroads. Deep in my gut, I knew I had a choice, just like before – the difference was this time I was aware of the consequences. Either I did everything in my power to stay in the here and now, or I would be imprisoned in my brain – again.*

Everything inside me wanted to go to sleep and go toward flowing into and with the warm, welcoming water. There are no words to adequately explain this extraordinary drive to let go and sleep; it was overwhelming and so much stronger than was humanly possible to resist. Then, another more powerful, compelling energy rose from deep within me. I needed to stay here because I had not completed all of my life purposes. I needed to teach people how to completely heal and enhance the brain, and everything else I have discovered. I needed to stay here to give people hope. I needed to stay here to continue my research and to teach others how to research the brain from the inside. I needed to be present for so many reasons, for so many purposes unfulfilled – some I did not even know about. I made a decision to stay here – to live in the present.

Immediately, I had an enormous gut sense to delve deeper into my precious inner awareness training while simultaneously focusing on – intensely being aware of outside objects: trees and leaves, signs, stoplights, people walking, etc. Of the utmost importance, I needed to consciously and continuously deepen my inner awareness while purposefully changing my outer focus so I would not become mesmerized by the outside objects and be drawn into that soft, warm, peaceful place and give up. Instantly, I made the decision and started delving deeper into my precious inner awareness training and focusing on outside objects as if my life depended on it.

While being driven home from a doctor's appointment, I called and explained the situation to a friend. I finished speaking and there was a pause. My friend's voice had a sense of urgency as he encouraged me to keep focusing on every single thing, even if I had to focus on each and every leaf. With a tear in my eye, I told him I would. The conversation ended, and I purposefully deepened my inner awareness while continually changing my outer focus; again, as if my life depended on it. After a few days, the overpowering need to sleep and the draw of the soft, warm, peaceful place dissipated.

In time, I healed from a nasty concussion, and there is no doubt the results could have been much worse. In the process of healing from the concussion, and more so afterwards; I spent a great deal of time thinking about both experiences. Twice, I was absolutely compelled to sleep and go into the warm, soft, peaceful place. The second time, I consciously chose to stay here – in the present. I wonder, could some people, during and right after they experience a stroke, brain trauma, etc., be helped by developing, or even better, delving deeper into their inner awareness training while purposely focusing on specific outer objects and persistently changing their outer focus? Would this technique help them not to be drawn into the soft, warm, peaceful place, or whatever their version is? I do not know, though I am looking forward to working with others to research my theory.

Although reflecting on all these experiences has been quite informative, I need to get back to the task at hand; healing from cancer. Throughout the rough chemo and radiation treatments, I am blessed by an abundance of support from fellow martial artists, my students and assistants, PFLAG family and friends, my family, and of course, my trusted friends and mentors. Some staff members at the hospital say they have never seen such an outpouring of help. People verbally tussle over who will drive me to the hospital, get me food, and workout with me – when I am up for it. Unfortunately, I am not able to workout like I want to; nevertheless, I keep on trying.

There is a Black Belt shave your head party which is a big hit. I am honored by the people who go bald and who cut their hair and donate it. My assistant, Robert Bowen proudly tells me he is going to keep his hair shaved for as long as I am bald. Every time I see bald heads, my spirit is lifted; their love and sacrifice encourages me more than they will ever know. There are also chemo parties where people bring all this great food to the infusion room, which is funny because I am trying not to throw up. At one party, we make so much noise that for the rest of the chemo treatments, I am relegated to the corner of the room, far away from other patients.

The outpouring of love and support is overwhelming, and I am not sure how to handle it all. Without hesitating, one of my friends says, "Cathy, don't you know how many people you have helped over the years! You have helped so many people, and now, they want to help you! Let Them!" Echoing in my mind are Ginny's loving words, "It's your time to receive." Consciously, I choose to open, accept, and receive love.

Right after the diagnosis I began having a crisis of faith. This the first time I have not been able to pray since I got down on my knees to get back on my feet in early sobriety. I am so pissed at God. Though, there is a very, very, very small part of me that knows Divine Source is not done with me.

After a rather challenging chemo and radiation regimen, the cancer goes into remission. I am beyond grateful for every person who helped me. The wonderful, caring doctors, nurses, and staff members, all my friends, colleagues, students, and family – there are way too many to mention.

In a routine check-up, a doctor, whom I have not met, tells me that for the rest of my life, I will be in excruciating pain throughout my entire body. I'm trying to comprehend what the heck he just said, but he continues talking about the cancer and the side effects of the treatments, then he leaves. A few minutes later, Dr. Kearsey walks into the room, and I ask her about what the other doctor said. She adamantly says, "Cathy, I know better than to tell *you, of all people,* something like that." We nod our heads and smile at each other. That doctor's words was his version of the "no's and never's" and "impossible's."

I develop a theory to deal with the agonizing pain. I believe if I keep working out and stretching, the pain will ease and one day, I will be free of pain. Equally important is the absolutely need to have hope; this powerful drive will keep me going when I do not want to. Little by little, I workout; it is the only thing that helps with the unbearable pain. My next appointment with Dr. Kearsey I share my microscopic progress and theory. She tells me the pain would be less if I was a couch potato, but that would be unhealthy. She encourages me to keep working out which I do.

I discover that there is a very fine line between working out too much and not enough. This is, and will be a very challenging formula to figure out. Months pass, and the pain is minutely better. My kicks are now three inches off the ground which is vastly different than being over my head before the cancer. Unfortunately, awake and asleep, tears run down my face from the constant, excruciating pain throughout my entire body. More time passes, and in the middle of a class at C.U., a student asks if I am sad. In a matter of fact manner, I say, "I am not sad. The tears are from the pain." I continue teaching, and what's interesting is that some people have a very difficult time dealing with my pain, which is funny because I'm the one in pain.

With a lot of time and effort, the pain very slowly decreases from a fourteen to an eleven. Although it feels like a reprieve, the agonizing pain is constant. I absolutely know not to focus on the pain as that will only increase it. Instead, I keep on working out, knowing it is simply a matter of time and effort before I am better than before. Thankfully, I have walked through my crisis of faith and have been praying for a while. I am closer than before with Divine Source.

On a very limited basis, I approach doctors and lay people

offering to teach and discuss my method – Brain Phoenix ™; as usual, it's all dead-end paths. A few of my family members want me to give up on my pursuit to teach my method. Though I understand their reasoning, *I absolutely know, way deep down inside, that if I give up, I will not fulfill one of the things I was placed on this earth to do: teach and speak about Brain Phoenix ™. My faith keeps me strong. I will keep getting better and complete all that I have been placed on this earth to do.*

39

A GLIMMER OF HOPE
LATE SUMMER
2007

I have a gut sense to travel to Oahu, Hawaii and explore the possibility of opening my two schools. Again, my main focus is my Brain Phoenix ™ school, to teach my method to people from around the world and also a Kung Fu School. The first place I plan on visiting is Tripler Army Hospital; it is in charge of fifty percent of all U.S. soldiers. The Department of Defense has ordered Tripler to find a solution to TBI and PTSD, which is a problem for some of the returning soldiers from the war. While driving to Tripler, I think about the almost eight years of approaching professionals, their organizations, and lay people about my method. *No one* has been willing to learn my method or discuss it in any detail. Said to say, I believe Tripler will be the most closed to my offer.

At the inspection gate, I am given directions to the Human Resource (HR) building, which is a separate building from the hospital. Opening the door to HR, I smile at the receptionist and sign in. A few minutes later, a woman calls my name and we walk to her office. While she's reading my cover letter and resume, she keeps glancing up at me. She re-reads the cover letter, but spends more time studying me. She finishes reading, leans forward, and intensely looks me square in the eye. She gathers her composure, then slowly gazes around her tiny office, leans over her desk and looks down the hall. Suddenly, she stands up and asks me to follow her.

We leave her office and swiftly walk down the hall, through the waiting room, and out the building. She stops at the curb and I think, for sure, I am being thrown out in no uncertain terms. Instead, she thoroughly scans the numerous parking lots that are filled with vehicles which surround the hospital and HR building. I too look around at the parking lots; no one is in sight for at least one-quarter of a mile. Quickly, she glances at my resume, looks up, leans in, and very quietly says, "We *really* need you here. But, I cannot hire you. There is no job code for what you do." Calmly, I say, "There is no job code because I am the one who developed my method." She understands, but still cannot hire me. Again, she strongly reiterates that they *really* need me here.

Next, she points to the massive pinkish, coral colored hospital and suggests, "Take your resume and find someone in the neurology unit. Maybe they can find a way to hire you because God knows we *really* need you here." She leans way in, and with an even quieter voice says, "I wish you well." She looks up, swiftly scans the area; then, hands back my resume and cover letter like it's a baton being passed in a race. In a flash, she is inside the building.

I am honored by this extraordinary woman and the tremendous courage it took to talk with me and point me in the right direction. I drive my rental car through parking lot after lot looking for a place to park. It is amazing how many parking lots and vehicles there are surrounding this immense hospital. A few minutes later, I find a spot.

Opening the door to Tripler Army Hospital I notice the hustle and bustle of people in and out of uniform moving with great purpose. In front of me is an info desk where I ask a young soldier for directions to the Neurology Unit. He smiles and politely says, "With all the construction projects, it will be more difficult than usual to find your way." He takes a deep breath and begins his detailed directions of a maze of corridors, elevators, and stairs that I will need to take to get around the different construction projects. To circumvent one project, I will have to go upstairs, down a hallway, turn right after the door, take the elevator down, take a right out the elevator, and down another hallway. The young soldier finishes his directions, smiles, and politely says, "I apologize for your inconvenience beforehand. People are quite friendly here; ask for help if you get lost. There are also signs which might help." I thank him for his abundance of directions and set off. After a few missteps, I arrive at the back entrance of the Neurology Unit. Quickly, I glance around. Up ahead and to my left is a door clearly marked "Joan the attack secretary;" she is the secretary to the chief neurologist at Tripler. I smile; if I can make it past her, I am in!

Confidently, I knock on the door. Joan opens the door and asks me to step in. Her office is tiny and filled with papers and filing cabinets. My first impression of Joan is she is very kind and a no-nonsense woman. I need to be very succinct when talking with her. I take a breath, and give my elevator speech while handing her my cover letter and resume. As Joan is reading, she is sizing me up, just like the woman from HR. She finishes reading and without missing a beat says, "We need you here. Please, do not move."

In the blink of an eye, she moves past me and out the door. I think about looking at where she went, but I do not dare. While waiting I read the different quotes, sayings, and cartoons taped on her door. I get up the gumption to glance at the direction Joan went, but I do not see anyone. I step back into her office and patiently wait. A few minutes later, she returns and says the chief neurologist is not able to see me now, but to call and make an appointment. I can tell Joan means what she says. I properly thank Joan for her time and tell her I will call.

I walk through Tripler and back to my car floating a few feet off the ground. I am elated; this is my first glimmer of hope! That day and the next few days, I approach other doctors, facilities, and lay people on Oahu. Even though the professionals and organizations cannot hire me, for the first time professionals are encouraging me to keep persevering in my endeavor to teach my method. As always, lay people are very supportive. I am energized by these meetings and the upcoming appointment with the chief neurologists at Tripler Army Hospital!

Though I spend the vast majority of my time approaching professionals and lay people, I also make the most of my time off. Before I traveled to Oahu, I studied travel books and mapped out the places I wanted to see. The first place I visit is the well hidden Spitting Cave. The entrance is a simple dirt pathway with a sign that is somewhat blocked by foliage. I get closer to the sign which is also warning that it's a treacherous area to hike, especially when wet. Fortunately, this is another gorgeous day in Hawaii. While hiking down the rocks and through the beautiful foliage, I see similar caution signs. I am grateful for all my training which is making my hike much easier. A few minutes later, I see the stunning blue water and awesome rock formation. Looking to my left, I see a wave crash into a giant rock wall. Almost immediately, the water looks like it is being spit out. A few seconds later, the ground trembles beneath my feet from the powerful explosion of water.

Next, I drive to the Dragon's Nostrils which has seven blowholes, including twin snorting nostrils. The view of the ocean as I hike down the lava hill is spectacular. Again, I am grateful for all my training; it's good to be sure footed. As I get close to the blowholes, I can feel a vibration under my feet from the fury of the ocean flowing under the lava. Every so often water and mist explodes through a few of the blowholes.

I meet two local kids and strike up a great conversation. They tell me they are going swimming in the Queen's Bath and offer to show me. We walk a short distance to a natural sort of rectangular pool in the lava. They say the Queen came here to take a bath and watch the Dragon's Nostrils and magnificent ocean. This place is stunning! As they are playing in the bath, I make a mental note. Either wear or have my bathing suit with me – always. I laugh as I say to myself; look at the palm of your hand and smack your forehead. Duh! Even with an intact brain, I can still goof up, but I am okay with making mistakes because I can learn from them.

I explore more of the island then return to the quiet youth hostel in downtown Waikiki. I love staying at hostels; I meet some exceptional people from all over the world. An added benefit is it only costs a little over thirty dollars a night to stay at this youth hostel. One of my friends helped me to make reservation at the youth hostel, and he graciously gave me his airline miles to travel to Oahu. I am so blessed; all my friends have huge hearts. The loving support and encouragement I have received to pursue my dreams is phenomenal. I go upstairs to my room, put on my bathing suit, and go for a relaxing swim which temporarily eases the excruciating pain a tiny, tiny bit. I love Hawaii with its warm weather and water, especially some of the quieter beaches. Early evening, I explore the downtown area and have a great meal. The food in Hawaii is excellent and the locals are so friendly.

Each day is a new adventure; I continue approaching doctors, nurses, etc. and lay people and they encourage me to keep persevering in my quest to teach my method. Again, I am pleasantly surprised by the outright support from professionals. Unfortunately, no one takes me up on my offer to teach or discuss my method.

The night before my appointment with the chief neurologist at Tripler, I plan the clothes I will wear and make sure everything is in order. The next day, I leave plenty of time to drive to Tripler, go through the inspection gate, find a parking spot, and walk through the vast maze to arrive at the Neurology Unit early.

Joan escorts me to the chief neurologist's office. I introduce myself and give my one minute plus summary of my method. Of course, I do not say that I was the one who had the TBI. I finish speaking and there is a very short pause, not the usual ten to fifteen seconds. He asks for a more detailed explanation of my method. I am stunned! In almost eight years, *no one* has asked for more information. Fortunately, I prayed beforehand to be given the words and they easily flow out my mouth. With ease, I explain more of my method and sketch some drawings. Next, I describe the people I want to work with: students must have a vested interest to learn my method and believe they will be completely healed. They must be willing and able to fully complete each step and my whole method. I want people who are highly motivated, and have a great attitude and integrity. I believe soldiers will do well and be more likely to fit into this group. That's one reason I want to work with soldiers.

The neurologist agrees and explains that most soldiers are highly motivated to work, especially if it will help them heal. I am impressed, and ask if I can ask some questions. He replies yes. I explain that I need a baseline neuro-psych test for every soldier with brain damage. He explains that they do not test every soldier because they do not have the personnel to give the test nor the money. I ask what they do. His eyes fall to the desk, and he shakes his head. Dejectedly, he looks up and says that they cannot do much. They give a few soldiers neuro-psych tests, but for the most part the soldiers clean up trash around the base. His voice trails off as he says he really wishes they could do more. I sense he is a kind, compassionate man and doctor who cares deeply about his patients. Suddenly, his whole energy changes, his face lights up, and there is a sparkle in his eyes as he asks how I would set up my program. *I am totally shocked! No professional has ever asked a single question, never mind two questions. Fortunately, I prayed beforehand to be given the words and they easily flow out my mouth.*

I explain that two-thirds of the class will be staff members with intact brains, and one-third will be people with disconnections in their brain. The main goal of people with intact brains is to learn my method, not to help the patients. The reason more people with intact brains are in the class is because I need people who, after receiving their teaching degree, will return to their state or other countries and teach others. I believe it will take people with disconnections in their brain a little longer to own my method then receive their teaching degree.

By simultaneously teaching people with intact brains and disconnections in their brain, I believe this will create a unique positive, healthy environment. People will experience the process of learning and healing within themselves and others. It is vital to be aware and listen to oneself and also the different experiences and words other people use to describe what is occurring within them – their inner awareness. These experiences will be crucial when they are teaching my method.

My experience is that progress is faster in a positive, healthy environment that encourages people rather than one which focuses on deficits. At times, a person with an intact brain will own a technique quicker than a person with disconnections in their brain and vice versa. Having a person ahead, whether it's someone with an intact brain or disconnections in their brain is a great incentive to push oneself in a healthy way. But, this isn't about competing with others, because the only place competition really resides is within one-self. When the individual succeeds, the group succeeds and vice versa. In addition, keeping one's ego right size, always having a student mind-set, being positive, encouraging, and taking responsibility for one-self, and doing all the work to get all the results is essential.

In the beginning, a class will be an hour long. The length of time will increase as student's strength and stamina improve. It is imperative that every student practice on their own and in groups when they are not in class. These practice times are vital for success because they allow students to integrate what they and others have become aware of which will further enhance their development. In addition, having or learning the skill of discipline to train on one's own will be crucial when they become teachers.

Throughout the conversation the doctor has been engaged and has treated me as a professional; however, when I finish speaking, his demeanor changes. He lowers his head, takes a deep breath, and reluctantly says that he would like to hire me, but his hands are tied. There is no job code for what I do. I change directions. I share how long and hard I have tried to break through the walls of the medical and research professionals and lay people. I have exhausted all options, and I do not know what to do. I explain that, over the years, people have suggested that I become a physical therapist, an occupational therapist, or a speech therapist, or a nurse. But, I know those professions do not have the power to make changes. He agrees. Recently people have asked me to become an M.D., and I am seriously thinking about it. However, I do not know if becoming a doctor would carry enough weight to make changes with the medical and research professionals? He answers with a definite, "No." I let out a sigh. His answer does not surprise me. I thank him for being honest, and for saving me a lot of money and many years of work. He smiles and nods his head. I ask if he has any other suggestions or is there anyone else I can talk with? He gives me the names of a few people at Tripler. Next, he commends me on what I am trying to accomplish. He also encourages me to keep persevering in my endeavor to teach my method and wishes me well. I approach the other professionals at Tripler. Long story short, people cannot hire me because there isn't a job code for what I do.

On the whole, my experience at Tripler Army Hospital has been very positive. People who work directly with patients: listened intently, were professional and respectful, and encouraged me to keep persevering. They share that there are so many people who need help. What a refreshing change, to be warmly greeted and treated with respect. It's funny; I thought Tripler would be the worst place to approach, but it turned out to be the best.

I continue looking for opportunities to teach and discuss my method on the island. Once again, the consistent comment of professionals is that they do not have the power to make decisions or changes. No one I have ever met has the power to make changes. I wonder; who has the power? I would really like to meet and talk with "them" and "they."

Professionally, my trip to Oahu has been very disappointing. On the other hand, I have met so many wonderful people with huge hearts and whose energy matched their words. I have also had great personal experiences. I have seen a lunar eclipse on the beach and was given a huge Royal Lei from people who knew the importance of what I was trying to do and encouraged me to keep persevering. The people of Oahu; professionals and lay people have encouraged me unlike anyone else in the world. They lift my spirit each time they ask me to keep persevering in my pursuit to teach my method. Mahalo!

My journey to teach, discuss, and speak about my method continues. I will share a few more stories that are quite informative. Here is the first. I have been trying to talk with the president of a rehabilitation hospital and my persistence pays off. I am given a few minutes of his time as he is walking to a meeting. Swiftly, I explain who I am, my method, and goals. Suddenly, he stops in the middle of the lobby and asks. "Are you going to steal our patients?" I am flabbergasted! He is serious – he is concerned about losing money! Quickly, I re-center myself and say, "No. I want to teach you, your staff, and your patients how to completely heal the brain, and everything I have discovered about the brain." He smiles and sarcastically thanks me for my time as he gently shows me to the door.

The next story is an event that has happened at different times with different people, they all have disconnections in their brain. Each person asks to *only* learn the 3 Day Inner Awareness Training to the Tan Tien. Again, I explain that my whole method needs to be completed, step by step, and that one technique will not heal their brain. Each person decides not to learn my whole method because they have been told over and over again that it is impossible to heal the brain. Next, they say a sentiment I have heard way too often. "Why try, it's impossible to heal the brain. Why try."

Years later, another person with disconnections in their brain insists that he *only* wants to learn the 3 Day Inner Awareness Training to the Tan Tien. Initially, I am against teaching him, but no one else wants to learn my whole method. With great reservations, I teach him the technique. After he practices this great technique, he shares how much it helped. I ask if he is ready to learn my whole method. His responds that he doesn't need any more help, can't I see all of his improvements? I patiently wait. Next, he shares all the things that are still so extraordinarily difficult to do because of the brain damage, especially the overwhelming exhaustion. Then, he states the very familiar response; he has accepted what the doctors and everyone else has told him over and over again; it's impossible to heal the brain. So why try. A sense of compassion wells within me. I am so thankful that I did not, and do not believe in the word impossible.

The last story is about people with different education levels ranging from; M.D.'s to high school graduates, they all have intact brains. Sarcastically, I am asked. "Will your method work for everyone?" Before I can speak, another person answers. "I bet she is going to say it will work for everyone." "Of course, she is going to say her method will work for everyone." I try to answer, but they continue to interrupt. When I am finally given the opportunity to speak, I calmly answer. "No, my method will not work for everyone, because people must believe they will be completely healed, they must be committed to and able to complete my whole method, and they must do all the work to get all the results. I am looking forward to finding out if method will work for others, and everything else it will positively do." For a very short period of time, I continue to speak, but nothing I say can penetrate their walls.

After this experience I make two decisions. First, I decide not to waste my time and energy talking with negative, disrespectful people, especially those who ask me to convince them, when they do not want to be persuaded. I firmly believe that people who respect themselves, respect others, and also people can disagree and do it respectfully and professionally. Second, people and organizations whose purpose is profit, prestige, and fame need not apply. Everything, absolutely everything is about my method – Brain Phoenix ™, helping others, and getting the message of hope about my method to people across the world; it is not about me, an individual, a group, or an organization.

All of my experiences have strongly demonstrated the need to make clear who I want as students, staff members, and the organizations that will work for and with me. My gut sense is in time, these requirements will continue to be fine tuned. As previously stated, right after I broke through the lock on and in my left temporal lobe and the automatic rebooting process, I was open to teach anyone; however, that has changed. Now, I want the best of the best. Professionals, organizations, and lay people with intact brains and disconnections in their brains must have a positive attitude, an excellent work ethic, be levelheaded, have integrity, be humble, and get along well with others. I am looking for people of character. They absolutely must take responsibility for themselves and their energy, and they must have common sense and utilize it. Students must believe they will be completely healed and they must be able to complete my whole method – do *all* the work, to get *all* the results. Students must be enthusiastic about learning my whole method and helping others. People must also be professional even if they are not a "professional." We will work diligently, and of course, have fun in a positive, healthy environment.

In addition, because of what I teach, I absolutely must be able to trust: my students, my staff, and the organizations who work for and with me. The interview process will be very thorough, and students will also go through in depth testing before, during, and after completing my whole method. I am most interested in students who will become teachers. To be clear a person does not have to be a teacher to become an instructor. After completing my whole method; then, receiving their teaching degree, my hope is they will return to their state or nation, and using the same high standards teach others. I am passionate about teaching students to become brain explorers; people who completely heal, enhance, explore, and research the brain, from inside the brain. I am looking forward to all the new positive and healthy discoveries, and growing, learning, thriving, missteps, and all of the successes.

I have made a change in the class distribution; fifty percent of students with intact brains and fifty percent of students with disconnections in their brain. Again, students with intact brains are not there to help the students with disconnections in their brain. My goal is to have great diversity in all of my classes, schools, and businesses; I want them to look like the United Nations. All of this will not happen overnight. This will sound very familiar; setting up, and running my schools and businesses will be a step by step process; it will be a journey not a destination. I am open and looking forward to having respectful, healthy, and constructive communication.

40

ANOTHER JOURNEY BEGINS AND THE POSSIBILITIES ARE LIMITLESS!

The solution to completely heal my brain from a TBI and enhance it better than before the accident was always inside me. My job was to delve deeper into my precious inner awareness training in order to develop my method Brain Phoenix ™. I am beyond grateful that my method unlocked the thick, blurry glass prison in my brain and fully reconnected me. I cherish my freedom and my ability to use my brain *at will*.

In my brain healing journey, I persevered *no matter what*, I learned to trust my gut, and turned missteps into great successes. Here is one accomplishment. I had lost the ability to write a sentence and every outside method I tried had utterly failed.

However, by utilizing my method, I not only wrote a sentence. Now, I have written this book, and my hope is it will open minds. The only place impossible resides is in the mind, but not in mine, and hopefully not in yours.

I believe the world is ready for a new era in healing, enhancing, and researching the brain – from inside the brain. I smile when I think of my next journey; teaching my whole method to people with intact brains and people with disconnections in their brain. I wonder in what other positive, healthy ways my whole method will be utilized, and all the good that will come from it. I believe the possibilities are limitless. Thank you for reading my story and if it has inspired you, I would appreciate your sharing the world-changing news with people all over the planet. Now there is a method to completely heal and enhance the brain better than before!

MOVING
FORWARD

I am open to respectful, healthy, and constructive communication, and looking forward to meeting positive transformation warriors. If you are interested in learning, discussing, and researching my whole method – Brain Phoenix ™, speaking engagements, and interviews please check out my website www.brainphoenix.com

BRAIN PHOENIX ™
A BASIC OUTLINE
TO COMPLETELY
HEAL AND
ENHANCE THE
BRAIN

Phase 1 of 3

*Baseline test, and testing throughout all 3 phases, including after completing my whole method.

*Always developing and delving deeper into the Inner Awareness Training.

– Simultaneously strengthening the body while positively challenging the brain. The foundation is internal and external martial art forms.

   – Simultaneous Brain Learning Method in every activity.

   – 4 Levels of Breathing, and balance – training and life.

   – Basic Meditation, and balance – training and life.

   – Continually change the simultaneous training.

   – The essential concepts of acupuncture, and also being aware while personally experiencing acupuncture.

   – Incorporating the Inner Awareness Training into every technique and activity.

*Future teachers; step by step, learn how to teach Brain Phoenix ™.

Phase 2 of 3

*Always delving deeper into the Inner Awareness Training in every technique and activity.

*Future teachers continue to, step by step, learn how to teach Brain Phoenix ™.

– Simultaneously strengthening the body while positively challenging the brain. The foundation is internal and external martial art forms.

    – Continually change the simultaneous training.

    – 3 Day Inner Awareness Training to the Tan Tien.

    – Able to do basic meditation while performing daily activities and training.

    – Advance meditation, and balance – training and life.

    – Second Connection – ming men: tan tien to ming men, play chi ping pong, clean up the pathway, slowly and consistently cultivate, invigorate, accelerate, and balance – the chi and training.

    – Circulate the chi in the centerline meridian of the upper body.

    – Circulate the chi through the limbs.

    – Circulate the chi in a continuous wave of energy through the body.

    – Invigorate the organs one at a time.

    – One meridian at a time: remove blockages, make connections, play chi ping pong, clean the pathway, slowly and consistently cultivate, invigorate, accelerate, and balance – the chi and training.

    – Mind-set; prepare to enter the Brain.

Phase 3 of 3

*Always delving deeper into the Inner Awareness Training in every technique and activity.

– Simultaneously strengthening the body while positively challenging the brain. The foundation is internal and external martial art forms.

– Continually change the simultaneous training.

– Decision; the brain is just another organ to be invigorated, healed, and enhanced.

– People with disconnections in the brain re-circulate the chi in the head meridians – in the healthy hemisphere or specific healthy area; one meridian at a time. People with intact brains re-circulate chi in the head meridians; one meridian at a time.

– Enter the brain.

– Invigorate the brain organ; people with disconnections in the brain invigorate only the healthy hemisphere or specific healthy area. People with intact brains invigorate the entire brain organ.

– Be aware and follow synapses in the healthy part of the brain.

– Move to specific, smaller healthy area of the brain; be aware and follow synapses.

– The automatic synapse reconnecting process and Internal Brain Mapping Technique.

– Area of the brain with the most damage, find the lock and the precise area with the deepest valley.

– Break through the lock; the Automatic Re-booting Process.

– Enhance the brain.

*Future teachers continue to learn how to teach Brain Phoenix ™, and upon completion of training to be a teacher, they receive their teaching degree.

www.ingramcontent.com/pod-product-compliance
Lightning Source LLC
Chambersburg PA
CBHW062157270326
41930CB00009B/1562